Health Related Counseling
with Families of
Diverse Cultures

Recent Titles in
Contributions in Psychology

Classifying Reactions to Wrongdoing
R. Murray Thomas

Prevent, Repent, Reform, Revenge: A Study in Adolescent Moral Development
Ann C. Diver-Stamnes and R. Murray Thomas

Post-Soviet Perspectives on Russian Psychology
Vera Koltsova, Yuri Oleinik, Albert R. Gilgen, and Carol K. Gilgen, editors

Multicultural Counseling in a Divided and Traumatized Society
Joyce Hickson and Susan Kriegler

Cognitive Psychology in the Middle Ages
Simon Kemp

Adolescence: Biological and Psychosocial Perspectives
Benjamin B. Wolman

Soviet and American Psychology During World War II
Albert R. Gilgen, Carol K. Gilgen, Vera A. Koltsova, and Yuri N. Oleinik

Counseling the Inupiat Eskimo
Catherine Swan Reimer

Culturally Competent Family Therapy: A General Model
Shlomo Ariel

The Hyphenated American: The Hidden Injuries of Culture
John C. Papajohn

Brief Treatments for the Traumatized: A Project of the Green Cross Foundation
Charles R. Figley, editor

Counseling Refugees: A Psychosocial Approach to Innovative Multicultural
Interventions
Fred Bemak, Rita Chi-Ying Chung, and Paul B. Pedersen

HEALTH RELATED COUNSELING WITH FAMILIES OF DIVERSE CULTURES

Family, Health, and Cultural Competencies

Ruth P. Cox

Contributions in Psychology, Number 43
Paul Pedersen, Series Adviser

GREENWOOD PRESS
Westport, Connecticut · London

Library of Congress Cataloging-in-Publication Data

Cox, Ruth P., 1947–
  Health related counseling with families of diverse cultures : family, health, and cultural competencies / Ruth P. Cox.
    p. cm. — (Contributions in psychology, ISSN 0736-2714; no. 43)
  Includes bibliographical references and index.
  ISBN 0-313-31477-2 (alk. paper)
    1. Family—Health and hygiene—Cross-cultural studies. 2. Family counseling.
  3. Family social work. I. Title. II. Series.
  RC455.4.F3 C69   2003
  362.1′04256—dc21   2002069615

British Library Cataloguing in Publication Data is available.

Library of Congress Catalog Card Number: 2002069615
ISBN: 0-313-31477-2
ISSN: 0736-2714

First published in 2003

Greenwood Press, 88 Post Road West, Westport, CT 06881
An imprint of Greenwood Publishing Group, Inc.
www.greenwood.com

Printed in the United States of America

The paper used in this book complies with the
Permanent Paper Standard issued by the National
Information Standards Organization (Z39.48-1984).

10 9 8 7 6 5 4 3 2 1

Copyright Acknowledgment

The author and publisher gratefully acknowledge permission to excerpt material from
the following source:

Cox, R. P., & Davis, L. L. (1999). Family problem-solving: Measuring the elusive
concept. *Journal of Family Nursing,* 5(3), 332–360. Reprinted by permission of Sage
Publications, Inc.

This book is dedicated to all the families who have honored me by allowing me to be part of their lives. I humbly thank all my teachers, colleagues, and friends who have given me their time. I thank my parents and family for the spirit and creativity they helped develop.

Contents

Tables and Figures

FIGURES

Series Foreword

In most of the world's cultures, the individual family member cannot be "healthy" unless the family is also healthy. Any problem influencing the family will also affect the individual members of that family. This family-centered approach to understanding and defining health is new and unfamiliar for most Westernized societies where individualism is the primary orientation. With the shift in demographic, social, economic, political, and military balance toward non-Western cultures it is essential to learn the "new rules" of collectivism and familial focused thinking. Cox presents encyclopedic coverage of the literature about families and health both across cultures and within specified cultures and then builds her own model on that solid foundation of research.

The purpose of this book is to integrate the family perspective in health care within a broad perspective of social and cultural systems that link families and individuals. The volume helps the reader understand the family in its sociocultural context, integrate theory and practice of health care for the family, and influence the effectiveness of families through appropriate health care interventions. The reader is carefully guided from an individualistic toward a family-centered perspective as an increasingly viable alternative mode of health care.

The chapters unfold from this conceptual starting point to review the different and changing definitions of the family as they develop. The theories and concepts that explain the family dynamics of health care are presented and discussed as they apply differently across sociocultural contexts. Although this book builds on the published literature and provides an empirical foundation for Cox's own model of family health care, Cox also "bumps up against the system" to suggest a variety of changes in family health care in a gentle nudge toward new approaches.

There are several features of this book that make it an ideal textbook. First, the conceptual ideas are described in itemized lists of features for each perspective. Second, there are numerous tables and figures that provide a visual picture of family functioning to clarify otherwise abstract ideas. Third, the assumptions behind each perspective are clearly identified. Fourth, the "points for counseling" are identified at the end of each chapter to demonstrate how this information can be applied. Fifth, a case study at the end of the book integrates Cox's own model in the context of a particular family.

The Greenwood Press Contributions in Psychology book series in which this book appears includes a long list of psychological issues in society. The series includes books on identity, culture shock, moral development, and other controversial applications of psychology to social issues. This book is consistent with the other books in this series by demonstrating the importance of rethinking the collectivistic and familial orientation as an alternative to prevailing individualism. This book will prepare the reader for the future in a global context where the family in its traditional and re-invented aspects will have a more influential role.

Paul Pedersen
Visiting Professor, University of Hawaii, Department of Psychology
Professor Emeritus, Syracuse University

Preface

Although it has always been known that families are the life of any society, more attention over the past decades has been given to families and their effect on health. Everyone grows up in a family of one kind or another—there can be no disputing that fact! Most individuals can describe the surroundings, the physical environment that was their playground for those growing-up years. What is often more elusive, not as clear, is the cultural, ethnic, and spiritual impact of those growing-up years in a particular family, community, society, and country. What part did family, community, society, country, play in the development of the individual and family? What are the hopes, dreams, biases, values that were created in the individual through his or her family? What is the continued interaction between all the players? How does this continued interaction over time affect individual and family health in society? How does society respond to the health care needs of families? Who makes the decisions in how a family responds to and receives health care? What medications are family members taking? What views and understandings do clinicians who work with families need to have in order to provide appropriate, gender and sexual identity-sensitive, culturally competent care?

The purpose of this book is to provide knowledge with an epistemological view that will help answer these questions. Although some progress has been made in integrating a family perspective in the U.S. health care system, most health care practice arenas continue to focus almost exclusively on the individual. This narrow perspective has critical limitations and fails to acknowledge the substantial effect families have on the health behaviors of their individual members. Furthermore, the modern view held by the present health care system fails to take into account the contribution that families can make to their own health care. This book's main purpose is to widen the health care perspective by providing a foundational view that incorporates both the family and the multiple systems with which they interact as resources for health. The purpose of this volume is to provide a foundation in the concepts of health-related counseling with families of diverse cultures; to learn how these concepts are used in clinical practice and during and after disasters; to see how these concepts drive political decisions at the local, state, and federal level; and to understand how these concepts drive family social policy or predict the future of family health care. An additional purpose of this book is to provide for clinicians, all in one source, the aforementioned information and information on common psychiatric medications, the types, ranges, uses, side effects, interactions with other drugs, effects on counseling, and collaboration needed among health professionals.

Due to the technological advancements, diversity, and complexity of our society, family health counseling is necessary to provide effective, efficient health care. It is my belief that clinicians must have a broad understanding of all the factors that affect individuals and families at all levels in order to provide effective culturally competent, collaborative care. Also, clinicians must have a theoretical framework or paradigm that guides their clinical practice with families. A postmodern view allows clinicians to enter into dialogical conversations and collaborative relationships with families. Thus, the client's voice can be heard over the clinician's thoughts about the client. This approach is based on the view that clients know the most about their situation and that when clinicians think they know more, interference results, with clients being unable to tell their stories and access their own resources.

This book expands the art and science of family health counseling into the new millennium. It will assist health and human service providers in their understanding of the critical ways in which family relationships, considered within their cultural/ethnic context, influence individual health behaviors. It does this by integrating theory, practice, and research with families from various family and counseling disciplines. This book makes the cognitive connections among epistimological views, theory, and clinical practice. This book was created as a textbook to be used by health care clinicians who want to question their continued seduction into linear, modern thinking. The text is for those who want to engage in and apply postmodern ideas to their present health care practice.

The book is appropriate for both undergraduate and graduate students who want a foundation in working with families within a multisystem paradigm. The text is suitable for students in counseling, marriage and family therapy, nursing, social work, family psychology, pastoral counseling, and family primary care physicians. The text provides readers an opportunity to broaden and expand their thinking in a reflexive, recursive manner.

Health Related Counseling with Families of Diverse Cultures: Families, Health, and Cultural Competencies is organized so that it can be used in its entirety for a course in family health counseling. Another alternative approach is to use Chapters 1, 2, 4, and 5 early in the curriculum as foundational knowledge. Chapter 2 contains all the material concerning family development over the life span, the components of family health, and family structure and process. If students are already familiar with this content, they can then become more involved with other chapters in the book. Then, as they begin their clinical practice, students can be exposed to Chapters 3, 6, 7, and 8 as a foundation for clinical practice. A third alternative is to use this book as a reference text or as an adjunct to other textbooks that address specific specialities.

The book is divided into eight chapters. At the end of each chapter is a section called Counseling Points, which alerts the reader to ideas from the chapter that will effect clinical practice. Chapter 8 is a case study that shows how material from the book is integrated into actual clinical practice with the Belcher family. Chapter 1, "Introduction: The Individual–Family Connection," lays a foundation for the connection between individuals and the families in which they grow up. Highlighted is the discussion of the family as the place where individuals are socialized and learn health behaviors. The family's role in society is discussed. This discussion leads to the family's role in the health of our nation. The leading health indicators and objectives of *Healthy People 2010* are identified. An important component of health care is deciding when clinicians need to be involved with families. This is discussed in the Family Health Care View Section, with a guide to when to assemble the family for care. The chapter ends with a discussion and identification of functional and dysfunctional family characteristics.

Chapter 2, "Family Development, Caregiving, and Functioning Over the Life Span," addresses family development over the life span, the components of family health, and family structure and process. Highlighted is the connection between the stages of the family life cycle and health concerns and health promotion needs. A concise table with each stage of the life cycle puts these concepts into perspective. Of interest is the discussion of two family life cycles, the adoptive family life cycle and the foster family life cycle. Chapter co-author Ken Farr, an advanced clinical practitioner in geriatric psychiatric/mental health nursing, expounds on the life cycle of the aging family. This is of interest as society begins to age and there is an increase in the number of persons of advanced age living in families.

Chapter 3, "Theories and Concepts: How to Understand Families and Health," presents a conceptual model for family health counseling. Along with this, a model for clinical practice is shown and its application to clinical practice is discussed. The historical evolution of family treatment is addressed along with some of the obstacles to family treatment in our present day health care system. I summarize several theories or concepts that direct clinical practice and family problem solving. Of interest are examples of the application of each theory or concept to clinical practice. Clinicians will be interested in the table with psychometric properties of thirteen instruments concerning problem solving that can be used in clinical practice. How clinicians can work with families using a reflecting team is discussed. A real-life example of this is shown in Chapter 4 with the Hispanic/Mexican case study.

Chapter 4, "Sociocultural Influences on the Family and Family Health," discusses and explicates many of the sociocultural influences on family health. Key concepts of culture, race, ethnicity, and social class are explored in the context of the family and our society. Emphasis is given to the interaction of culture and social class and its effect on family health. Sylvia London and her colleagues from the National University of Mexico provide an example of the interplay of culture and family work in their case study. Specific outcome evaluation of their work is given verbatim by the family.

Chapter 5, "Family Health Issues," defines family health, and factors influencing family functioning and health are discussed. Family health promotion and ecosystem factors affecting this are explored. Highlighted are examples of questions that clinicians can use to explore family health, health promotion, and illness and disease within families. This chapter examines family health policy and how social policy impacts lesbian and gay families.

Chapter 6, "Family Assessment Tools," describes and gives examples of assessment tools that can be used with families. An in-depth genogram is shown that incorporates family history, culture, health, and relationships within the family. Clinically relevant working hypotheses are given about family patterns for categories of the genogram and ecomap. Of interest for clinicians is the section on medications commonly used with mental health problems. This section identifies the different categories of psychiatric drugs, gives examples and usual dosages for each drug, side effects, identifies interactions between psychiatric drugs and other medications, and explicates common concerns for clinicians. The impact of psychiatric medications on the counseling process is explored and the need for collaborations and referrals is discussed.

Chapter 7, "Family Health Counseling, Counseling in Disasters, Health Interventions, and Reimbursement with Families of Diverse Cultures," expands on material in the preceding chapters and puts it in a clinical context. The chapter presents the components of family health counseling, assessment, treatment plan, family interventions, and evaluation. It discusses how to develop a therapeutic relationship with multicultural families and the importance of supervision and training when working with families. Legal and ethical issues when working with families are discussed as well as the politics of gender in clinical practice. Skills for transcultural family counseling are identified. Examples of their clinical application are given in the case study in Chapter 8. A research focus is discussed in that there is a need for evidence-based treatments when working with families. Reimbursement issues are addressed as these vary from state to state. Next, family counseling in disasters is explored with possible resources during a disaster identified. In conclusion, examples are given of family and community resources that can be utilized after a disaster.

This book is meant to be a catalyst, in a friendly enough manner (according to the Chilean biologist, Humberto Maturana), to bump against the system and broaden the thinking of those who read this book, and to effect collaborative, recursive clinical practice with families. I encourage all who read the book to write me with your ideas and thoughts about the book and its impact on clinical practice with families. My greatest hope is that this book will impact you enough so that you join with families in a manner in which you are not the expert and you can co-create self-agency within families so that they can accomplish their goals!

1

Introduction
The Individual–Family Connection

Ruth P. Cox

The family is the earliest social institution in which "a lifetime of physical and mental health or lack thereof" is established (Hanson & Boyd, 1996, 16). Research outcomes support a connection between health and the family in that health and illness behaviors are learned within the context of the family (Pratt, 1976). When a family member experiences health problems, this affects the whole family (Friedman, 1986; 1998; Gilliss, 1993; Greenberg, Greenley, McKee, Brown, & Griffin-Francell, 1993; Seaburn, 2001). The family also is a significant factor in the health and well-being of individuals (Gilliss, 1993). Family theoreticians suggest the following: families affect an individual's health, and an individual's health and health practices affect the family (Doherty, 1985; Doherty & Campbell 1988; Doherty & McCubbin, 1985); health care is more effective when it includes the family rather than the individual alone (Gilliss & Davis, 1993); and promotion, maintenance, and restoration of the family's health are important to society's survival (K. Anderson & Tomlinson, 1992).

There is a growing recognition that health crises are critical events in the life of a family (Hanson & Boyd, 1996). When such crises occur, the mental and physical health of family members can deteriorate along with deterioration in the family's functioning. However, families also have opportunities to increase their adaptive capacity and mental health during a crisis. Family counselors can provide supportive interventions to help them during these critical events.

Interest in the study, treatment, and evaluation of families has increased in all health professions. The traditional disciplines of nursing, medicine, social work, and psychiatry have begun to offer course work (i.e., in family theory, family interviewing, and family therapy) that is related more to the context of their treatment system—the family. In the health care system today, professionals work more frequently with clients and their families to solve problems. This family problem solving, especially for health-related problems, occurs within the larger context of the family's culture. This book is built on the premise that clients in hospitals, clinics, or professional offices benefit more from assistance that is *family-centered care* (Freidman, 1986) and culturally competent (Giger & Davidhizar, 1995). Over the past four decades, family health counselors have shifted from seeing and treating the individual as a single unit to viewing an individual within the context of his or her family system (Friedman, 1986, 1998). The focus is on providing the clinician with a knowledge base for holistically understanding and assessing families from diverse cultures. The outcome of assessing factors influencing family functioning and health within a cultural context provides a therapy framework leading to constructive, culturally competent changes at the family system level.

FAMILY AS THE UNIT OF SOCIALIZATION AND LEARNING HEALTH BEHAVIORS

Through the generations and in all cultures, the family has been the unit of socialization for members of a society (G. Lee, 1982). The family is the institution for childrearing, the provision of emotional care, love, and affection, and the transference of cultural values and beliefs. An individual's hopes, attitudes, and aspirations are influenced by their early years within the family. The Rameys have been studying the influence of early family life on early childhood growth and development for more than twenty-five years (Ramey & Ramey, 2000). They suggested that "the early years count—a lot" (p. 2). To fulfill their potential, all individuals need to have "early positive learning experiences followed by equally strong opportunities later, in schools, at home, and in their 'free-time' activities" (p. 2).

Ramey and Ramey reported findings of a recent study, the Abecedarian Project in North Carolina, in which children had early childhood education and parenting support. These children, when compared with children who did not receive early childhood education and parental support, showed higher levels of performance on measures of intelligence, language, reading, math, and real-world indicators such as lower rates of grade repetition and placement in special education. As young adults, they were more likely to go to college, to be fully employed, and to have delayed childbearing. Also, programs like Healthy Families America (U.S. Department of Justice, 2001) emphasize the importance of early years in the family. This program provides support for families with young children with the intent of preventing child abuse and providing a safe environment for the first years of life, those most critical for brain development.

A family is usually defined as two or more persons residing together, who share economic resources, are related by birth, marriage, or adoption, and who have a commitment to each other over time (Walsh, 1993). Even family pets may be considered as "members of a family" (Cox, 1993; Rosenkoetter, 1991). The family into which a person is born is referred to as the *family of origin* (Foley & Everett, 1981). The family that is created when a person leaves his or her family of origin to begin his or her own family is called the *nuclear family*. Individuals who have unresolved family-of-origin conflicts often carry these issues with them into their nuclear family. These unresolved problems can affect the healthiness of the nuclear family. For example, survivors of incest and sexual abuse in their family of origin often experience relational and/or marital problems in their nuclear family.

Families are where individuals learn lifelong attitudes and health behaviors (Cox, 1997). Tinkham and Voorhies (1984) suggested that families provide the critical resource for delivering efficacious health services. Behaviors of one family member, whether healthy/unhealthy–adaptive/maladaptive, affect other members within the family unit as the family is a closely knit, interdependent network whose members mutually influence each other. There is such a strong relationship between family and the health status of individual family members that illness or problems in one family member will "'seep in' and affect the other family members and the whole system (the 'ripple effect')" (Friedman, 1998, p. 5).

FAMILY'S ROLE IN SOCIETY

As the family is the basic unit in society, it shapes and is shaped by the community and larger society in which it exists (Friedman, 1998). When considering family functions and tasks, it is clear that the healthier the family, the healthier the society. In establishing the nation's health, emphasis is placed on both health promotion and risk reduction. These activities are initiated within the family environment and are supported by different societal agencies, such as the school system and recreational agencies (i.e., community swimming pools). Thus, the family interacts with the society in which it exists and the health of the society is dependent on the actions of the family—a reciprocal effect. Family health behaviors are acted out within the context of not only the family, but also that of the larger community and society (Stanhope & Lancaster, 1996). In turn, the larger community and society are made up of and depend on the well-being and functioning of the family. Furthermore, family lifestyle and the environment interact with hereditary tendencies passed down throughout the family's generations. Thus, it is imperative that the family carry out its role of health promotion and reduction of health risk as an important approach to improving the health of the society in which it exists.

FAMILY HEALTH AND THE NATION—HEALTHY PEOPLE 2010

The United States has emphasized the importance of health promotion and disease prevention for improving the quality of family life. Three documents from the U.S. Department of Health and Human Services: *Healthy People: The Surgeon General's Report on Health Promotion and Disease Prevention* (1979); *Promoting Health/Preventing Disease: Objectives for the Nation*

(1980); and *Healthy People 2000: National Health Promotion and Disease Prevention Objectives* (1990) provided goals for the nation concerning health promotion for individuals and families. The newest document, *Healthy People 2010* (1998), builds on these initiatives over the past two decades.

The goals for *Healthy People 2010* (1998) are twofold: (a) increase quality and years of healthy life; and (b) eliminate health disparities. Ten leading health indicators (LHIs) have been identified that are the high priority areas for the nation's health. These LHIs will be used to evaluate public health progress over the next decade and will serve as a focal point to coordinate national health improvement efforts. The LHIs are listed here:

1. Physical activity
2. Overweight and obesity
3. Tobacco use
4. Substance abuse
5. Responsible sexual behavior
6. Mental health
7. Injury and violence
8. Environmental quality
9. Immunizations
10. Access to health care

Although these LHIs seem to be focused on the individual, the accomplishment of the objectives related to the LHIs will take place within the family setting—thus the importance of the family in meeting the nation's goals of *Healthy People 2010*.

The major objectives for the new century with examples for each include the following: (a) promote healthy behaviors (i.e., physical activity and fitness); (b) promote healthy and safe communities (i.e., environmental health, education, and community-based programs); (c) improve systems for personal and public health (i.e., access to quality health services, health communication); and (d) prevent and reduce diseases and disorders (i.e., cancer, diabetes, and mental disorders). Clinicians can use the LHIs and the four major objectives as areas to help focus their work with families regarding family health promotion.

FAMILY HEALTH CARE VIEW

Levels of Clinician Involvement

Doherty (1985), a family social scientist, suggested that it is important for families to be involved with clinicians during the health care experience. He identified a continuum for family involvement by health care providers. This is based on the clinician's expertise and needs of the family.

At Level 1, families are involved only when needed for practical or legal reasons. For example, the family must sign for a child to be involved in counseling and/or testing or a procedure for a child who is under the age to sign him or herself. The clinician's expertise is minimal for explaining and gathering consent and/or assent.

At Level 2, families are involved when information and advice is needed through regular contact with the family. For example, the counselor may advise the family on the progress of a child who is in treatment through regular weekly meeting or in a "family week" that is often done in treatment centers. The clinician's expertise is that of being knowledgeable and accurate about the information that is given to the family.

At Level 3, families are involved to assist clinicians and provide support when dealing with emotional reactions to stressful situations that the clinician knows will occur based on his or her knowledge of normal family development. For example, bereavement and grief over the death of a child. The clinician's expertise involves empowering and assisting family members in discussing their reactions and supporting them in their coping efforts. The clinician's expertise allows the care to be individualized to the particular needs of the family, so it will look different depending on the stress event and the needs of that family.

At Level 4, families are involved when systemic family assessment is needed due to the health problem and interventions being planned. For example, a husband, who has several other health problems, is being brought home after an automobile accident that has left him a paraplegic. The clinician's expertise involves understanding family systems, being aware of his or her own family system, and understanding larger systems in which the family and health care providers operate. The clinician may be involved in coordination and collaboration of care with the family. This level of family care requires more knowledge and skill and often the clinician has a graduate degree.

At Level 5, the most complex level of care, families are involved when the health care problem is difficult and/or complex and often there are strongly opposing views on what the solution should be. For example, a mother wants her child to return home from a treatment facility, whereas the husband and siblings want the child to stay in the rehabilitation center for further care that they believe cannot be given at home. The clinician's expertise requires advanced knowledge of family systems and patterns of dysfunctional interaction and skill in working with dysfunctional families. The clinician at this level is a specialist in mental health care to whom the family has been referred or who is consulting with other health care providers who are providing the care. The level of care requires the ability to hold a family conference, assess family functioning and mediate the decision-making problem-solving process.

When to Assemble the Family for Care

Although different levels of family care lead to different types of family involvement, there also are times when the family, as a group, needs to assemble for health care problem solving. Doherty (1985) provided guidelines to assist health care providers to know when to assemble the family as a whole. Table 1.1 identifies when to assemble the family when making health care decisions. The top section of the table deals with who in the family is seen, whereas the bottom section gives examples of the type of health care problems for which the person or family is seen.

The following situations are indications for a family assessment:

- A family is experiencing emotional, physical, and/or spiritual suffering/disruption caused by a family crisis (i.e., sudden illness, injury, or death).
- A family is experiencing emotional, physical, and/or spiritual suffering/disruption caused by a developmental milestone (i.e., birth, marriage, child leaving home).
- A family defines the problem as a family issue and there is motivation for an assessment (i.e., impact of chronic illness on the family).
- A child or adolescent is identified as having the problem (i.e., school behavior).
- The family is experiencing issues serious enough to jeopardize family relationships (i.e., child abuse, physical abuse).
- A family member is to be admitted to the hospital (i.e., for psychiatric treatment).
- A child is to be admitted to the hospital (Wright & Leahey, 2000).
- A family member is admitted initially for individual issues but with further assessment, the problem is defined as family related (Clarkin, Frances, & Moodie, 1979).
- A family breaks up and separation and child-care issues need to be decided (i.e., joint custody, child support, visitation; Wright & Leahey, 1994).

This information can assist clinicians in determining when to assemble the entire family, although they may have been dealing systemically with the family when only an individual is seen (Cox, 1994). Assembling the entire family is an opportunity for the clinician to perform both individual and family assessment simultaneously. This provides a context for the clinician to assess for serious risks such as suicide, homicide, and other serious illnesses in individual family members (Wright & Leahey, 1990).

FAMILY FUNCTIONAL/HEALTHY CHARACTERISTICS

A person's ability to deal with constant life changes and stress stems from experiences and skills learned in the family. Family and health characteristics have been identified that effect the development of competent, healthy individuals who are able to maintain a mentally healthy lifestyle (Beavers, 1977; Kelly, 1978). Table 1.2 specifies characteristics found in a healthy family.

How an individual applies those skills learned in his or her family of origin to manage life changes, determines the person's relative mental wellness. If the individual leaves the family of origin with healthy communication, high self-esteem, few unresolved issues, and a hopefulness about the world, his or her

Table 1.1.
When to Assemble the Family in Health Care

Generally see Client Alone	Family Conference Desirable		Family Conference Essential
Minor acute problems	Routine self-limiting problems	Treatment failure or regular recurrence of symptoms	Chronic illness
		Routine preventive educational care	Serious acute illness
			Psychosocial problems
			Lifestyle problems
			Death

Source: W. Doherty (1985). Family intervention in health care. *Family Relations, 34,* 129–137. Copyrighted by the National Council on Family Relations, 3989 Central Ave. NE, Suite 550, Minneapolis, MN 55421. Reprinted by permission.

Table 1.2.
Healthy Family Characteristics and Components

Characteristic	Component
1. Open system view	Events have many causes
	Many factors inside and outside affect the family system
	Need for each other in the family system & others outside the family
	Family system is flexible and open to interchange with its environment
2. Boundaries- Internal and External	Well defined internal with open external inter-system boundaries
	Appropriate touching occurs with others within & outside the family
	Family members interact face-to-face with one another
	Space for privacy in household as culturally appropriate
	Links to outside organizations-work, school, church, friends, community
3. Contextual clarity	Clear mulitigenerational lines
	Strong parental coalition with no parentification or scapegoating
	Maintain collaborative marital relationship/roles as culturally appropriate
	Oedipal/Electra issues resolved
	Communication is clear, congruent, honest, direct, and specific
4. Power	Within the parental diad or intergenerationally as culturally appropriate
	Delegated to children appropriate for age
	Clear role definition-members know and agree on their activities
	Agreement of position of each family member
	Not gender defined as culturally appropriate
	Well defined and respected procedural and relational rules
5. Encouragement of differentiation	Acceptance of differences as culturally appropriate
	Encourage expression of individual's ideas which differ from family's
	Emotional space made for each member of the family
	Member idiosyncrasies tolerated well
6. Affective issues	Members have empathy, warmth, respect, and caring for each other
	Feelings are encouraged to be discussed and attended to
	Amount of conflict is low/very low as culturally appropriate
	Resolution of conflict without loss of self-esteem/keep high self-esteem

**Table 1.2.
Continued**

7. Negotiation and task performance	Led by parents at family meetings with parents making final decisions
	Input from all members and outside resources as culturally appropriate
	Little amount of conflict
	No significant deviance in school, work, or relationships with others
	Responsibilities appropriate to developmental level
8. Transcendent values	Expect, prepare, and recover from loss
	Hopeful, positive outlook
	Atruistic toward others
	Concern for the environment
	Crisis dealt with appropriately
9. Spirituality	Members yearn for connection with a greater power than themselves
	A superior Being acts relationally for welfare & beneficial change
10. Health measures	Family history of health
	No alcohol or substance abuse
	Regular exercise, recreation, and a healthy diet
	Health maintenance and wellness checkups
	Absence from dangerous activities
	No significant health problems

relationships in the nuclear family have greater potential to be healthy. If the individual prematurely or suddenly leaves his or her family of origin in an effort to deal with unresolved family conflict or leaves at the appropriate time but with unresolved issues (i.e., incest or abuse), relationships within the nuclear family may be adversely affected and result in unhealthy relationships. Relationships with and within the family of origin may also be adversely affected.

Lewis, Beavers, Gossett, and Philips (1976) also composed a list of characteristics of a healthy family system that include the following:

1. Affiliative vs. oppositional attitude toward encounters
2. Respect for own and others' subjective worldview
3. Openness in communication vs. distancing, obscuring, and confusion mechanisms

4. Firm parental alliance without competing parent–child coalition

5. An understanding of human motivation as varied and complex versus a simplistic, linear, or controlling orientation.

6. Spontaneity versus rigid stereotyped interactions.

7. High levels of initiative versus passivity.

8. Encouragement of unique versus bland human characteristics (p. 202).

FAMILY PROBLEMATIC CHARACTERISTICS

Families with difficulties often produce individuals with inadequate relationship skills, physical health problems, mental health problems, behavior disorders, troubled relationships, or who exhibit antisocial behaviors, borderline personality disorders, or psychotic disorders (see Table 1.3; Beavers, 1977; Kelly, 1978).

Individuals who come from unhealthy families or who leave their family of origin with unresolved issues and carry these issues and problems into their nuclear family, may seek out a person with whom they can work out these unresolved issues or past relationship problems (Dicks, 1967; Scharff & Scharff, 1991). These unresolved issues and past problems may surface again in nuclear family relationships in similar ways to those experienced in the family of origin. For example, adult children from alcoholic family systems may transport the unresolved problems and the same difficult relationship patterns from their family of origin into their nuclear family relationships.

In assessing a family, the clinician must discern whether the problem lies only within the nuclear family, is part of an unresolved issue from the family of origin, or a combination of both. Clinicians may ask the following type of questions to determine whether the present problem has originated in the nuclear family, has its origins in the family of origin, or both: "You tell me that you are drinking a lot now. Did you see this happening when you were growing up or did you decide *now* it would be a way to handle your problems?" (the nuclear family); "When you were growing up, did you see drinking going on in your family or your parent's family?" (family of origin); "Am I understanding you correctly that your father drank when he was upset with your mother, and that you also drink when you are upset with your wife?" (both).

COUNSELING POINTS

- The family is the origin of early influence on its individual members and their health.
- The family is instrumental in understanding individual and family relationships, values, and beliefs.
- A society and nation is only as healthy as its families' health.
- Clinicians and families must be collaborative for the best health outcomes.
- Specific family and health characteristics create healthy, competent individuals.

Table 1.3.
Characteristics and Components of Problem Families

Characteristic	Component
1. Open system view	Absent-members need others under certain circumstances
	Believe there are specific causes for events and search for answers
	Strive to do well as culturally appropriate
	Blame the outside system for problems within the family
very troubled families:	Family may appear rigid or chaotic/disordered
	Family trusts the internal family more than external community agencies
2. Boundaries-	May appear clear-when under pressure members turn inward and
Internal and External	solidify boundaries or outward into the community, i.e., legal problems
	Intra-system interaction is restricted and distancing often prevalent
	Links to community may be present but disrupt under pressure
very troubled families:	May appear rigid with few links to society as culturally appropriate
	May be diffuse with family business spilling into the environment with possible contact with police
	Interpersonal boundaries may be rigid with resultant family violence
	Interpersonal boundaries may be diffuse resulting in the whole family responding to outside input as culturally appropriate
	Family members operate at developmental stages lower than for age
	Society links can be tentative/mistrustful with limited input from larger society
3. Contextual clarity	Parental coalition present but weak/ineffective as undermined by other coalitions, parentificaton, and/or scapegoating
	Marital relationship is often secondary to parental relationship
	Parents may reach across generational boundaries for comfort and support often forming unhealthy triangles as culturally appropriate
	Child who is "triangled" is often the family symptom bearer-presents with mental disorders, physical illnesses, or delinquent behavior

(continued)

Table 1.3.
Continued

	Oedipal/Electra issues are unresolved due to stifling and stereotyping of sexual expression as culturally appropriate
	Overt or covert incestuous situations may be present and intergenerational
	Communication may be clear at times but expressed with fear, guilt, or anger
very troubled families:	Communication: not clear, honest, or specific; incongruence between verbal and nonverbal occurs with double-bind communications; failure to attend to messages (disqualifying) occurs through silence, ignoring, evasiveness, or changing the subject; anger expressed through hitting and other forms of abuse
	Incestuous relationships may be sanctioned
	Child is seen as "the problem" in the family or the family would be fine
	Parental relationship has dissolved
	Marital relationship has dissolved
4. Power	Power and love may be confused as members are controlled through overt/covert coercion or through "oughts" / "shoulds" that are often gender-stereotyped as culturally appropriate
	Parents deal with children by doing the "right thing" through discipline or coercion as culturally appropriate
	Children learn power through manipulation rather than learning responsibility
	Children are given power that is developmentally and age inappropriate

Table 1.3.
Continued

	Roles are defined by gender or beliefs about the person
	Family behaves as if they are being judged for rightness of actions and
	beliefs as culturally appropriate
very troubled families:	Power may be diffuse and does not come from parents
	Family members are loyal to a leader rather than societal norms
	Corporal punishment is used by parents as culturally appropriate
	Roles are assigned regardless of gender or developmental readiness
5. Encouragement of	Not found - children are expected to adhere to family norms and power
differentiation	struggles are constant as culturally appropriate
	Constant suppression of feelings and creativity as culturally appropriate
	Children may stay at home into adulthood or leave early
	(pseudoautonomy) as culturally appropriate
	Children at early age may be mother or father in or out of wedlock
	Children may engage in unsafe practices, i.e., drug dealer, prostitution
very troubled families:	Autonomy discouraged
	Differences not tolerated but family will identify one member as
	"different" and the cause of the family trouble
	Violent actions occur often with police involvement
	Family members are often incarcerated
	Children are mother or father multiple times, in or out of wedlock, and
	are not involved with nor supporting their family
	Children leave home to live an unsafe life style, i.e., drug dealer,
	prostitution

(continued)

**Table 1.3.
Continued**

6. Affective issues	Depression, anxiety, and anger with resulting conflict expressed openly
	with anger, or repressed with submission to "oughts" and "shoulds"
	Little empathy or genuine caring shown
	Large amount of conflict over rules and family/societal/cultural norms
	Caring is controlling rather than growth producing
	Members self-esteem is low
	Self-esteem of identified client is very low
very troubled families:	Self-esteem is low & hate, loneliness, and hopelessness predominate
	With diffuse boundaries, affective tone is exaggerated, members react
	inappropriately to threats or one member's difficulties, and police are
	often involved with the family
	With rigid boundaries, affective tone is restricted, depressed, and
	despairing undue attention (confusing, smothering, and rejecting) is
	shown to one member
7. Negotiation & task	Accomplished by coercion as parents cannot agree on who does what
performance	Children may often be part of the decision making process
	No family meetings but work of family is accomplished
	Tasks are age inappropriate
	Children often have school problems regarding grades and/or behavior
	Parents often lose their job, are jobless, or are in low paying jobs
	Difficulty in negotiating with other family and extended family members
	Family members operate at developmental stages lower than for age
	Family developmental tasks behind developmental stage
very troubled families:	Negotiation not accomplished as culturally appropriate
	Tasks vary widely and are probably age inappropriate
	Family members operate at developmental stage several stages lower
	than for age

Table 1.3.
Continued

	Family developmental tasks not accomplished successfully
	With diffuse boundaries, conflict may be overt, constant, an
	unresolved with legal interventions
	With rigid boundaries, conflict is denied, not commented on
	unresolved both inside and outside the family
8. Transcendent values	Hope, caring, and altruism are lacking
	Change and loss accepted with enormous pain, anger, and frustration
	Martyrdom may be a stance both inside and outside the family
	Look to the future for difficulties rather than being hopeful
	Crisis causes family instability with long recovery time
very troubled families:	Absent or found only in one or two members who are more
	disconnected from the family unit
	Inability to deal with loss or differences
	Cynical, hopeless outlook
	Family has repeat offenders in the legal system who have not
	responded to rehabilitation
	Family members may belong to a gang, cult, or special antisocial group
	Crisis can cause family to spiral into chaos
9. Spirituality	Family members may feel connected to a higher power but do not act
	out these values within their family relationships
	Members question the impact a superior Being has on the family
very troubled families:	See themselves as the determinator of their lives
	Superior Being has no impact on family members or their lives
	No ability to enjoy each moment of their life
	No inner peace to be found outside themselves as culturally appropriate

(continued)

Table 1.3.
Continued

10. Health measures

Excessive use of alcohol, prescription drugs, and other drugs to relieve

pain of each day

Psycho-physiological illnesses (i.e., headaches, ulcers, obesity, eating

disorders)

Meet basic health needs but no health promotion or wellness activities

Attempts recreation and exercise but often conflict when making plans

Sometimes excessive anger level leads to family violence, child and

elder abuse, driving at excessive speeds, road rage, or running away

very troubled families:

Can be serious physical illness, usually in one member

Delay of necessary medical treatment for acute and chronic illnesses

Child/elder abuse that necessitates medical treatment

Use of alternative health treatments when modern medicine is needed

as culturally appropriate

Family violence that leads to police and/or legal intervention

2

Family Development, Caregiving, and Functioning Over the Life Span

Ruth P. Cox and Ken Farr

CHANGING FAMILY DEMOGRAPHICS

Today there are many different family compositions and no single definition fits all families. Clinicians working with families must expect to see many different groups defining themselves as a "family." Comonly occurring family compositions have been identified by Duvall and Miller (1985). (See Table 2.1 for a list and definition of these.) Also, there are multiple other types of family compositions emerging in our society today (see Table 2.2 for a list and definition). There are other possible family members such as best friends, neighbor children, and nieces and nephews (Hanson, 2001).

Over the past several decades, major changes have taken place in American families that have lead to the changes in how families look—their composition. Trends reported by the U.S. Bureau of the Census (1989a, 1989b, 1989c, 1989d; 1991a, 1991b; 1992a, 1992b, 1992c, 1992d) indicate increases in divorce, re-marriage, age at first marriage, working women, and delays and declines in childbearing. Families are smaller than they were in the 1980s and more likely to be composed of a single parent or multiple wage earners, require child-care assistance, and contain stepchildren (see Table 2.3). These trends mean families must face more transitions today as people form, dissolve, and reform families several times over individual lifetimes.

FAMILY LIFE CYCLE: DEVELOPMENTAL STAGES, TASKS, AND HEALTH ISSUES

Intact Family Life Cycle: Stages of Family Development

Over time, the family evolves and changes while accomplishing the functions and tasks of the family. The idea of family *life cycle* rests on the assumption

Table 2.1.
Family Compositions

Type	Definition
1. Nuclear	Two-generational, married couple and children by birth or adoption
	Single career: husband breadwinner with wife at home; wife breadwinner with husband at home
	Dual career: both spouses employed when married-wife's career interrupted due to child care/wife starts career after children enter school
2. Nuclear dyad	Husband and wife, childless (cannot have children), with one or both employed
3. Extended-multiple generations	Nuclear family plus other relatives whether by birth, adoption, or marriage
4. Alternative	Adults of a single generation or a combination of adults and children who live together without the social sanction of marriage (i.e., communal arrangement)
	Roommates who are heterosexual or gay/lesbian couple/s
5. Single parent	One adult due to death, separation, divorce, or abandonment along with children
	Single adult with adopted child:
	Parent working
	Parent not working, supported by government funds, family, or life insurance and savings
6. Blended/step [reconstituted]	Remarriage of spouse/s where parents, stepparents, children, and stepchildren live together
	Single career or dual career

Source: Duvall and Miller (1985).

that families have a great degree of interdependence (McGoldrich & Carter, 1982). Table 2.4 identifies the stages of family development including the transition stage of family development from the typology described by McGoldrick, Heiman, and Carter (1993) and the eight stages of development as described by Duvall (1971; Duvall & Miller, 1985). This approach seeks to describe change over time in interactions and relationships within the family. It is based on the observation that families are long-lived groups with a natural history that must be assessed if the family is to be fully and accurately understood (Duvall & Miller, 1985). However, this approach does not cover nonfamily aspects of individuals over time or events affecting the individual that do not impinge on the lives of other family members (Aldous, 1996).

Family life over time is understood as a series of stages with transitions between stages, but with breaks that give each stage distinctive characteristics (Klein & White, 1996). The idea of stages rests on the assumption that families are forced to change each time members are added or subtracted or each time the oldest child engages in new developmental tasks. For example, there are changes in roles, marital relationships, child rearing, parental care taking, and discipline as time goes by and the family ages, moving from one stage to another. All families will move through each time period or stage in their own unique way. When children are preschool age the family has one structure, another structure when children reach adolescence and the parents are in the prime of their life, and yet another structure when children leave home and the parents are on their own and/or caring for their elderly parents. Each different stage requires different tasks and skills and proposes different health issues related to health promotion and health problems that the family must face.

In contemporary society, diverse family groups will experience stages of development at different points in time and often several stages at the same time. For example, a blended family, involved with placing young adults into society and the developmental tasks of this stage, may again re-enter the childbearing stage with its different developmental tasks when the couple chooses to have other children together. Families who, at the same time, are dealing with several stages and the family developmental tasks related to each stage are families at risk who may need more support to successfully negotiate the changes and stages they will experience.

Family developmental theory is based on general features of the everyday life of a family with predictable changes and growth. Clinicians, however, need to be aware that this approach does not address situational or non-normative stressors (unusual events). It can be "criticized for its assumption of homogeneity (its lack of adequate attention to family diversity), its middle-class bias, its assumption of stability within each stage, and its lack of explanation of the processes that occur between stages that allow families to change" (Friedman, 1998, p. 112). Also, this approach does not deal with cultural diversity as a whole nor cultural diversity within a family multigenerationally (McGoldrick et al., 1993).

Developmental theory fails to deal with the issue of a maturity that includes interdependence as "the reality of continuing connection is lost or relegated to the background" (p. 413). Sibling relationships, as an example of the longest relationships that may occur, are not discussed. Spiritual growth of individuals within the family and the family as a unit is not discussed. Clinicians must adjust to the fact that Duvall and Miller's model alone does not incorporate the varied family forms that exist in society today. Neither does it include stages

Table 2.2.
Family Compositions: Emerging Family Structures

Family Type	Composition
Single adult	Living alone, usually with a career, who may or may not desire to marry
Middle-aged/ aging couple	Husband as provider, wife at home - children have been launched into college, career, or marriage
Kin network	Nuclear households or unmarried members living in close geographical proximity and operating within a reciprocal system of exchange of goods and services
Second-career	Wife entering the workforce when children are in school or have left the parental home
Institutional	Children in orphanages, residential school, or correctional institutions
Binuclear	Divorced parents assuming joint custody and co-parenting responsibilities for a minor child; the child is part of a family system consisting of two nuclear households
Commune	Monogamous- household of more than one monogamous couple with children, sharing common facilities, resources, and appliances; socialization of the child is a group activity
	Group marriage- household of adults/offspring known as one family- adults are married to each other and all parent the children; usually develops a status system- leaders believed to have charisma
Intentional community	Individuals and families who want to live in close geographical proximity to one another by design
Unmarried parent- child	Usually mother and child where marriage is not desired/possible
Unmarried couple- child	Usually a common-law marriage with the child their biological offspring or informally adopted
Dyadic nuclear	Husband and wife chose not to have children; one or both are employed
Homosexual	Homosexual couple, male or female, living together with or without children; children may be informally or legally adopted; may or may not be legally married/recognized

Table 2.2.
Continued

Cohabiting retired couple	Unmarried retired couple living together, usually because financial hardship would result if they married (retirement benefits would decrease)

Table 2.3.
Family Demographics[a]

Type of Family	1970	1990	2000
All families [b]	51.2	64.5	71.7
Married with children (%)	49	36.9	34
Married without children (%)	37.1	41.7	42.8
Single-parent families (%)			
Female 88%	5.7	10.2	9.7
Male 12%	0.07	1.8	2.7
Same-sex households (%)	2	2	
Unmarried couples (cohabitation)	520,000	3 million	
People living alone (%)	20	20	
Births to single mothers (%)	11	27	

[a]Figures given as percentages of total number of households.
[b]Figures given in millions.
Source: U.S. Bureau of the Census (1990). *Current population reports*, Series P-20, No. 128.

nor tasks related to divorced families, remarried families, nor domestic partner relationships.

Intact Family Life Cycle: Stage Developmental Tasks

As described in the previous section, the family can be viewed in terms of the different life-cycle stages throughout its development. Each stage in the

Table 2.4.
Stages of Family Development

Stage	Definition
Transition Stage [a]	Between families/Unattached young adult (individuals in their late teens/twenties; financially independent; physically left their family of origin; not begun their own family)
Stage 1 [b]	Beginning families (married couple)
Stage 2 [b]	Early childbearing families (oldest child age thirty months)
Stage 3 [b]	Families with preschool children (oldest child age two-and-one-half to five years)
Stage 4 [b]	Families with school children (oldest child age six to thirteen years)
Stage 5 [b]	Families with teenagers (oldest child thirteen to twenty years)
Stage 6 [b]	Launching center families (children leaving home)
Stage 7 [b]	Families of middle years (empty nest through retirement)
Stage 8 [b]	Family in retirement and old age (retirement to death of both spouses)

Source: Adapted from: [a]McGoldrick, Heiman, and Carter (1993) and [b]Duvall (1971); Duvall and Miller (1985)

family life cycle is thought of as a space of relative stability that is qualitatively and quantitatively distinct (Mederer & Hill, 1983). What occurs during each of the family life-cycle stages is generally referred to as developmental tasks for each stage. These family developmental tasks are to be accomplished within each stage for the family to feel satisfied during that stage and for optimum preparation for the next stage of family development. Table 2.5 identifies each stage, starting with the Transition Stage: Between Families, with the tasks for that stage. These family stage-specific tasks deal with meeting biological requirements, cultural imperatives, and the family's own unique values and aspirations (Duvall, 1977; Klein & White, 1996).

Family developmental tasks are created through the circular interchange between the family striving as a unit to meet individual family member's needs and the individual family member striving to meet his or her individual needs.

Table 2.5.
Family Life-Cycle Stages with Developmental Tasks, Health Concerns, and Health Promotion Needs

Family Stage [a]	Developmental Tasks [a]	Health Concerns [b]	Health-Promotion Needs [b]
Transition stage:	Separating from family of origin	Family planning/birth control	Health protective practices (i.e.,
Between families	Developing intimate peer relationships	Sexually transmitted disease	avoid drugs, alcohol, tobacco)
	Establishing work and financial	Accidents	Engage in safe sexual practices
	independence	Suicide	Obtain adequate sleep, nutrition,
		Mental health problems related to	exercise
		separation from family of origin	Preventive dental care
		Premarital counseling	Preventive medical exams
			Cultural and spiritual
			development

(continued)

Table 2.5.
Continued

Stage 1: Beginning families	Establishing a mutually satisfying marriage (i.e., who does what and when) and money management	Marital and sexual role adjustment	Adequate time for marital adjustment before pregnancy
		Family planning	Family planning education and counseling
	Relating harmoniously to the kin network	Communication-intellectual and emotional	Prenatal family education and counseling (i.e., physical health of
	Planning a family-parenthood-adjusting to pregnancy	Preparation for parenthood	mother), family adjustment to new family member
	Establishing a workable philosophy of life as a couple	Adapting patterns of sexual relationships to pregnancy	Establishing ways of interacting with friends and community organizations
		Prenatal care	Cultural and spiritual development

Stage 2: Early childbearing families	Postpartum health	Family-centered maternity education
Setting up the young family as a stable unit (integration of new baby)	Postnatal classes	Family planning counseling
Reconciling developmental tasks and needs of various family members (i.e., where authority lies, costs, home life)	Follow-up home visits	Cooperative extended family member adjustments
Learning cues baby expresses to make needs known	Infant and well baby care	Education of when and from whom to accept help
Maintaining a satisfying marital relationship	Early recognition of health problems	Education of when to depend on own strengths and inner resources
Expanding relationships with extended family by adding parenting and grand-parenting roles	Immunizations	Strong marital relationship
Fitting into community life	Safety measures	Healthy parent/child relationships
Reworking a family philosophy of life	Sibling relationships	Cultural and spiritual development
	Family interactions-parental and marital	
	Child-care facilities for working mothers	

(continued)

Table 2.5.
Continued

Stage 3: Families with preschool children	Meeting family members needs for adequate housing, space, privacy, safety	Children-accidents, falls, burns, frequent communicable diseases, fire drills with meeting place	Family health education directed at healthy lifestyle areas of
	Socializing children	Family-psychosocial needs and marital relationship	• smoking
	Integrating new child members while still meeting needs of other children	Sibling rivalry	• alcohol and drug misuse
	Maintaining healthy relationships in the family (marital and parent/child) and outside the family (extended family/community)	Family planning	• sexuality
		Growth and development needs	• safety
	Learning to separate from child	Discipline	• diet and nutrition
	Meeting predictable and unexpected costs of family life with small children	Home safety	• exercise
	Creating and maintaining effective communication within the family	Family communication	• social support
	Tapping resources and serving needs outside the family	Adequate child care facilities	• stress management
	Reworking family philosophies of life		Cultural and spiritual development

Stage 4: Families with school-aged children	Socializing the children, promoting school achievement, fostering healthy peer relations of children, and capacity for work enjoyment Maintaining a satisfying marital relationship, promoting open communication Meeting physical health needs Finding fulfillment in rearing the next generation while "letting the child go" Providing for children's activity and parents' privacy Keeping financially solvent Feeling close to extended relatives Participating in life outside the family Testing/retesting family life philosophies	Possible child problems (i.e., visual, hearing, speech defects, learning problems, behavior disturbances, epilepsy, cerebral palsy, mental retardation, cancer, orthopedic conditions) Dental problems Child abuse/neglect Substance abuse Communicable diseases Marital relationship problems Childrearing practices	Yearly well examinations Health care screenings Support counseling for families with children with problems/disabilities Cultural and spiritual development

(continued)

Table 2.5.
Continued

| Stage 5: Families with teenagers | -Balancing of freedom with responsibility as teenagers mature & become more autonomous
Learning to accept rejection without deserting the child
Communicating openly between parents, children, and grandparents
Couple learning to build a new life
Maintaining ethical and moral standards
Providing facilities for widely different needs
Discussing money with teenagers
Keeping in touch with relatives
Reworking/maintaining a life philosophy | Communication problems with parent and teenager
Discipline and power struggles with parent and teenager
Drug/alcohol misuse
Birth control
Teenage pregnancy
Accidents
Athletic injuries | Discuss risk factors related to age
Exercise
Recreational activities
Support counseling for marital relationship and parent/teenager relationship
Teenage pregnancy prevention strategies
• family planning services
• sexuality counseling/ education
• after school leisure activities
• educational opportunities
Cultural and spiritual development |

Stage 6: Launching center families	Learning to build a new life (marital couple) without children continues	Parent/young adult communication problems	General health promotion regarding:
	Rearranging physical facilities/resources	Role-transitional problems for husband and wife	• exercise
	Meeting family expenses	Care of and assistance to aging parents	• nutrition
	Coming to terms with themselves as husband and wife	Emergence of chronic health problems and/or predisposing factors, such as:	• breast/neck/testicular exam
	Maintaining open systems of communication within and outside the family	• high cholesterol levels	• report mouth sores
	Widening the family circle through release of young adult children with appropriate rituals and assistance	• obesity	• seat belts
	Recruitment of new members through marriage of children	• high blood pressure	• stress reduction
	Assisting aging and ill parents of couple	Menopause for women and men	• obtain dental exam/prophylaxis
		Effects of prolonged drinking, smoking, and dietary practices	Family planning for adolescents and young adults
			Cultural and spiritual development

(continued)

Table 2.5.
Continued

Stage 7: Families of middle years	Learning to build a new life for the marital couple continues	Filial care of and assistance to aging parents leading to physical, emotional, marital and financial caregiver strain (usually daughters)	Need for wellness lifestyle
	Providing a health-promoting environment	Grandparent and in-law roles	Report postmenopausal bleeding
	Maintaining a pleasant/comfortable home environment	Emergence of chronic illness continues	Dental prophylaxis
	Assuring financial security- later years	Effects of children leaving home	Cultivation of leisure-time activities and interests
	Drawing closer together as a couple	Parents' sense of adequacy in their parental and work roles	Preventive health screening
	Maintaining contact with grown children's families	"Plateau phenomenon" related to work leading to stress and health problems	Preventive health exams (i.e., stool guaiac, mammography, sigmoidscopy)
	Keeping in touch with brothers' and sisters' families and with aging parents	Adjustment to physiological changes for women and men	Preventive strategies re: middle-age crisis and job-related stress
	Participating in community life beyond the family		Renegotiation of marital system as a dyad rather than parents
	Reaffirming the values of life that have real meaning		Relationship building to prevent "marital blahs" and "comfortable rut"
			Cultural and spiritual development

Stage 8: Family in retirement and old age	Learning to adjust/accept the dependent role	Declining health status: physical, mental, and cognitive	Adjustment to loss of work role
	Closing family home/adapting to aging	Mobility or self-care limitation	Adjustment to a reduced income and to economic dependency
	Establishing comfortable house	Psychophysiological vulnerabilities	Preparation for loved one s death
	Finding a satisfying home for the later years	of aging, such as:	Preparation for possible move to assisted living facility and later, an institutional setting
	Adjusting to retirement and income status	• diminished physical vigor	Injury prevention
	Nurturing each other as husband and wife	• gastrointestinal changes	Nutrition counseling
	Facing bereavement and widowhood	• depression	Exercise and recreational activities
	Caring for elderly relatives	• confusion	Teaching safe use of medicines
	Maintaining contact with children and grandchildren	• fewer financial resources	Use of preventive services
	Keeping an interest in people outside the family	• social isolation	Cultural and spiritual development
	Finding meanings in life - life review and integration	• loneliness	Use of community resources (i.e., Senior Center; Homemakers Services; Geriatric Day Care)
		• loss of loved ones	
		Retirement	
		Death of spouse	
		Adjustment to environmental changes	
		Nutritional deficiencies	

[a]Duvall (1971); Duvall and Miller (1985); McGoldrick et al. (1993)
[b]Friedman (1998)

Expectations from the community in which the family resides, cultural and spiritual factors, and the wider society also create family tasks. Although not discussed specifically in Duvall's model, these expectations will look different from culture to culture and from spiritual resource to spiritual resource.

Intact Family Life Cycle: Health Concerns and Health Promotion Needs

The stages of family development approach seeks to describe change over time in interactions and relationships within the family. Duvall's original work did not explicitly address health concerns and issues. However, as the family develops over time, common health concerns and health promotion needs arise within each stage of family development. These concerns and needs will develop within the cultural/ethnic context of the family, side by side with the general development of the family unit—an interweaving of these, each one affecting the other. To be aware of all factors that affect the family and individuals within the family, these factors must be considered within the holistic view of the family.

When a counselor or other health professional is dealing with a family, the health concerns and health promotion needs at that point in time must be taken into account for the best possible outcome of the family unit. Therefore, along with the family development stages and the tasks for each stage, Table 2.5 identifies the health concerns and health promotion needs for each stage. These include both family and individual concerns and needs related to physical, mental, psychosocial, and spiritual health that will be specific to the family's culture or ethnic heritage.

Intact Family Life Cycle: Impact of Illness and Disability on the Developmental Stages

Given the assumption of reciprocity, it is clear that serious illness or long-term disability of a family member affects the family and its functioning, while reciprocally, the family and its members simultaneously affect the course and character of the illness or disability. This in turn influences the development of the family and its individual members, especially the ill or disabled member. Often, lower family functioning and thus a delay in mastery of family developmental tasks occurs when the family is overloaded with both developmental demands or stressors and situational demands or stressors.

Several factors affect the extent to which the family developmental tasks and individual developmental tasks for that stage are affected. These factors include the family's life cycle stage, which family member is ill or disabled, and the formal and informal resources of the family. Clinicians can assess and evaluate the impact of the illness or disability on the family and individual developmental tasks accomplishment by comparing the developmental tasks of the appropriate family life-cycle stage with the family's actual behavior (Friedman, 1998).

Separation: The In-Between Stage of Development

Separation is a transition between living in an organized family household to a family reorganized in divorce or significant other break-up, and possible remarriage/new significant other. Not all separations end in divorce or break-up. Major developmental family-role transitions occur in this stage, as well as divorce and remarriage/new significant other. During these times, the family will undergo adjustment, restructuring, and consolidation (Stanhope & Lancaster, 1996). Ahrons and Rodgers (1987) suggested that during this time, family members work to regain or maintain themes that the family values. Developmental transition phases are listed here:

PRE-SEPARATION

Gradual emotional separation

Continue to enact public/social roles

Avoid exposing state of the relationship to the public

Initiator usually experiences guilt

Assentor usually experiences anger

EARLY SEPARATION

State of emotional and social anomie

Emotional ambivalence as feelings vacillate

Ambiguity of separation itself

Status of family undefined

MID-SEPARATION

Emotional distress still felt

Faced with a deficit in structure with two separate households

Realignment of family member relationships

Conflict between meeting own needs and children's needs

Convert anxieties into "other-directed" anger

Restructure tasks to meet children's health and nutritional needs—outside support possible

Try to form a co-parenting relationship

Seek support from friends, relatives, neighbors, and so on

LATE SEPARATION

Old patterns replaced by new ones as family reorganizes

Trial-and-error time for meeting needs

Power struggles of the marriage become more exaggerated

Reassessment of economic condition of family and friendships

Create a sense of family for all family members

Clinicians can use these developmental transition phases, with strategies for each phase, as a guide in assessing, directing, and evaluating the family's transition during this phase of the family life cycle.

Divorced Families Life Cycle

There are a variety of alternative living arrangements and marital status within society (see Tables 2.1 and 2.2). Of note is the high rate of divorce. Saluter and Lugaila (1998), in their review of census data, reported that the "currently divorced population is the fastest growing marital status category" (p. 1). Today, divorces are so common (almost 50% of all marriages end in divorce) that the event is being viewed as a "normative transition" (Friedman, 1998, p. 138). "It is becoming increasingly apparent that divorce should be viewed not as a discrete event but as part of a series of family transitions and changes in family relationships" (Hetherington, Law, & O'Connor, 1993, p. 208). Young adults most often experience divorce, with a mean age of thirty-four (Hanson & Boyd, 1996). Divorce is higher for African Americans and Hispanics than for Whites. Recently, there has been an increase in couples over sixty years old who were married for many years before divorce. About two thirds of all divorces involve one or more toddlers, preschoolers, or school-age children (Hanson & Boyd, 1996).

In 1996, divorced persons represented 10% of adults age eighteen and over, an increase from 3% in 1970. Between 1970 and 1996 in the United States, the proportion of children living with one parent increased from 12% to 28% (Wright & Leahey, 2000). Of these children 86% live with their mother. There was an increase in the number of children living with their fathers—9% in 1970 and 14% in 1996. In 1996, the percent of children living with one parent varied by race: 57% Blacks, 32% Hispanics, 27% Whites.

The single-parent divorced family is under great pressure as they must accomplish the same developmental tasks as a two-parent family, but without all the same resources. The remaining family members are burdened as they must compensate with increased effort to accomplish all the family tasks, such as support, childrearing, companionship, and gender role modeling for the children. Hill (1986) suggested that "the differences in paths of development of single-parent and two-parent families are seen primarily, not in stages encountered, but in the number, timing and length of the critical transitions experienced" (p. 28).

From their research with thirty employed single parents, Quinn and Allen (1989) indicated that these women were challenged in managing shortages of time, money, and energy. These parents had serious concerns about meeting societal and family expectations of being single and living in a family with two parents. There was a clear double bind between behaviors necessary to manage a family alone and those behaviors that might attract another husband. These women might need assistance in planning responses in a variety of situations as a single mother.

Carter and McGoldrick (1989; 1999) conceptualized divorce as a disruption in the family life cycle. This disruption can have a wide variance of reaction for individual family members ranging from enhanced competence to clinical levels of problem behavior (Hetherington, et al., 1993). "The response to any family transition will depend both on what precedes and follows it" (p. 208). Divorce may incite a series of adverse factors, such as economic decline, parenting stress, and physical and psychological dysfunction in family members. On the other hand, "divorce may be an escape from conflict and abuse in an unsatisfying marital relationship, provide the possibility of healthier relationships, and/or be an opportunity for personal growth and differentiation" (p. 209).

Divorce cannot be separated from its contextual environment. Thus, the following factors must be considered in understanding divorce and the effects it has on individual family members over time and multigenerationally: (a) social and historical context, (b) cultural/ethnic context, (c) changing dynamics within the family and multiple generations, (d) individual ontogenic characteristics of parent and child, and (e) influences outside the family (i.e., extended family, peer relationships, work situation, and societal systems of education, mental health, law, spirituality, and welfare).

Divorce is a major disruptive force that complicates the complexity of the developmental tasks the family is experiencing. Subsequent stages are affected so that every stage after the divorce must be viewed within the context of both that stage itself and the aftermath of the divorce. Family research has found that it takes a minimum of two years for the family to re-establish itself after a divorce. If this does occur, the normal family developmental processes can continue (McGoldrick, et al., 1993). Carter and McGoldrick (1999) summarized Ahrons' (1980) research and writings on the adjustment process that families go through. Table 2.6 outlines the pre- and post-divorce process within divorced families. This includes the emotional processes that are a prerequisite to each of the developmental issues for each of the phases.

The impact of the divorce on the family varies depending on what stage the family is in when the divorce occurs. Other factors also contribute to the effect, such as cultural, ethnic, social, spiritual, and economic factors. Divorce is the least disruptive during the early stages of the family life cycle as there are

Table 2.6.
Stages of the Divorce Family Life Cycle

Phase	Emotional Process of Transition - Prerequisite Attitude	Developmental Issues
DIVORCE		
1. The decision to divorce	Acceptance of inability to resolve marital tensions sufficiently to continue relationship	Acceptance of one's own part in the failure of the marriage
2. Planning the break up of the system	Supporting viable arrangements for all parts of the system	a. Working cooperatively on problems of custody, visitation, finances b. Dealing with extended family about the divorce
3. Separation	A. Willingness to continue cooperative co-parental relationship B. Work on resolution of attachment to spouse	a. Mourning loss of intact family b. Restructuring marital/parent-child relationships; adapting to living apart c. Realignment of relationships with extended family; staying connected with spouse's extended family
4. The divorce	More work on emotional divorce: Overcoming hurt, anger, guilt, etc.	a. Mourning loss of intact family: giving up fantasies of reunion b. Retrieval of hopes, dreams, expectations from the marriage c. Staying connected with extended families

POST-DIVORCE		
1. Single-parent family (custodial household or primary residence)	Willingness to maintain contact with ex-spouse and support contact of children with ex-spouse and his/her family	a. Making flexible visitation arrangements with ex-spouse and his/her family
		b. Rebuilding own financial resources
		c. Rebuilding own social network
2. Single-parent (Non-custodial)	Willingness to maintain parental contact with ex-spouse and support custodial parent s relationship with children	a. Finding ways to continue effective parenting relationship with children
		b. Maintaining financial responsibilities to ex-spouse and children
		c. Rebuilding own social network

Source: From Carter and McGoldrick (1999). *The expanded family life cycle: Individual, family and social perspectives* (3rd ed). Published by Allyn and Bacon, Boston, MA. Copyright © 1999 by Pearson Education. Reprinted by permission of the publisher.

Table 2.7.
Effects of Divorce on Children and Parents

Age	Effect of Divorce
Young children	Initially most affected: regress developmentally; behavior problems
	Single parenthood difficult for the mother
	Father often loses connection with children
School-age children	Long-term impact more profound—not old enough to deal effectively with the divorce yet knows what is occurring
Adolescents	Compounds the problems of adolescence
	Developmental tasks and the family life cycle are initially delayed
Adult children	Less profoundly affected as are more autonomous
	May end up supporting one parent during the divorce
Older adult children	Most profoundly traumatizing to the divorced partners, likened unto the death of a partner

fewer people involved (perhaps there are no children in the family), fewer established traditions, and fewer couple-based social ties (Peck & Manocharian, 1988). The family is most at risk for divorce and the impact is greatest during the third and fourth stages when there are preschool and school-age children in the family. Table 2.7 identifies the effect that divorce can have on children and parents at different ages.

Clinicians can use Tables 2.6 and 2.7 as a guide in assessing, guiding, and evaluating the family's transition during this phase of the family life cycle.

Remarried Family Formation/Stepparent Families Life Cycle

An increase in stepfamilies in North America in the recent decade has occurred as two thirds to three fourths of those who divorce remarry (Wright & Leahey, 2000). Therefore, by the time they reach sixteen years of age, an increasing number of children are living in stepfamilies (Hanson & Boyd, 1996). Most of these children live with their biological mother and stepfather rather than stepmother and biological father. Berger (1998) reported that one in three Americans is a part of a stepfamily.

Remarriage, because it is a disruptive transitional process, slows the family's movement through, and completion of, family developmental tasks. As with divorced families, remarried families take a minimum of two to three years before a new structure allows the family to move forward developmentally. In Table 2.8 Carter and McGoldrick (1999) suggest a developmental outline of the remarried family—the steps involved, prerequisite attitudes, and developmental issues. The family's emotional process in the transition to remarriage typically involves struggling with the following:

- Fears about investment in a new relationship
- Each partner's fears
- Fears of the children involved
- Reactions of the children, extended family members, and ex-spouses
- Ambiguousness of the new family organization
- Increased arousal of parental guilt and concern over the children
- Positive and/or negative rearousal of the old attachment to the ex-spouse

Stepfamilies are unique in that they have different issues than the nuclear families from whence they came (Goldenberg & Goldenberg, 1998). Uninformed clinicians may unknowingly increase rather than decrease family tension if they communicate that stepfamilies should be like their biological families. Visher and Visher (1996) suggested differences between stepfamilies and nuclear families and the therapeutic implications for working with stepfamilies (see Table 2.9).

Ahrons and Rodgers (1987) suggested that it is possible to have *bi-nuclear families*. This term indicates a different type of stepfamily structure without inferring anything about the quality or nature of the ex-spouses' relationship. These can be joint-custody families or families in which the relationship between the ex-spouses is friendly. From their work, they have developed the following relationship types:

- Perfect pals: spouses whose previous marriage has not destroyed their friendship.
- Cooperative colleagues: not good friends but worked well together for the children.
- Angry associates: spouses are furious with each other.
- Fiery foes: spouses are outraged with each other.
- Dissolved duos: spouses no longer have any contact with each other.

Ahrons (1998) supported a normative process model for working with divorced families rather than focusing on pathology or dysfunction. It is important to keep in mind that it is a complex situation when working with stepfamilies, as each family brings with it its own set of circumstances and resources. There are no "simple answers to whether on-going contact with fathers following divorce is beneficial or detrimental for children" (Healy, Malley, & Stewart, 1990, p. 531).

Mills (1984) suggested stepfamily developmental tasks that could be used when working with families. These tasks can be used as a guide by clinicians

Table 2.8.
Remarried Family Formation: A Developmental Outline

Steps	Prerequisite attitude	Developmental Issues
1. Entering the new relationship	Recovery from loss of first marriage (adequate "emotional divorce")	Recommitment to marriage and to forming a family with readiness to deal with the complexity and ambiguity
2. Conceptualizing and planning new marriage and family	Accepting one's own fears and those of new spouse and children about remarriage and forming a stepfamily Accepting need for time and patience for adjustment to complexity and ambiguity of the following: a. Multiple new roles b. Boundaries: space, time, membership, and authority c. Affective issues: guilt, loyalty conflicts, desire for mutuality, unresolvable hurts	a. Work on openness in the new relationships to avoid pseudomutuality b. Plan for maintenance of cooperative coparental relationships with ex-spouses c. Plan to help children deal with fears, loyalty conflicts, and membership in two systems d. Realignment of relationships with extended family to include new spouse and children e. Plan maintenance of connections for children with extended family of ex-spouse(s)

| 3. Remarriage and reconstitution of family | Final resolution of attachment to previous spouse and ideal of "intact" family; acceptance of a different model of family with permeable boundaries | a. Restructuring family boundaries to allow for inclusion of new spouse-stepparent
b. Realignment of relationships throughout subsystems to permit interweaving of several systems
c. Making room for relationships of all children with biological (noncustodial) parents, grandparents, and other extended family
d. Sharing memories and histories to enhance stepfamily integration |

Note: Variation on a developmental schema presented by Random, Schlesinger, and Derdeyn (1979).

Source: From Carter and McGoldrick (1999). *The expanded family life cycle: Individual, family and social perspectives* (3rd ed.). Published by Allyn and Bacon, Boston, MA. Copyright © May 13, 2002 by Pearson Education. Reprinted/adapted by permission of the publisher.

Table 2.9.
Stepfamily Differences and Therapeutic Implications

Differences	Therapeutic Interventions
Different structural characteristics	Evaluate family using stepfamily norms
Little or no family loyalty	Initially seeing the family together may be unproductive
Before integration the family reacts to transitional stresses	First focus is on transitional adjustment, not intrapsychic processes
Society compares stepfamilies negatively to nuclear families	Basic need for acceptance and validation as a family unit
Long integration period with predictable stages	Stage of family development is very important in the assessment of whom to see
No breakdown of family homeostasis as equilibrium has not been established	With normalization and education, stability can emerge
Complicated "supra-family system"	Complications need to be addressed
Many losses for all individuals	Grief work may be necessary
Pre-existing parent–child coalitions	Developing a secure couple relationship is paramount
Solid couple relationship does not signify good stepparent–stepchild relationship	Step-relationships take special attention separate from couple relationship
Different balance of power	Stepparents have little power. Discipline needs to be handled by the biological parent
Less family control due to influential parent elsewhere or in memory	Appropriate control can be fostered to lessen the anxiety engendered by helplessness
Children have more than two parenting figures	Think in terms of a "parenting coalition"
Ambiguous family boundaries	These losses and stresses may require attention
Initially no family history	Members need to share past history and develop new family rituals
Emotional climate is tense and unexpected	Empathy with other family members is to be encouraged by understanding needs not being met: to be loved and appreciated, to belong, to have control over one's life

Table 2.10.
Stepfamily Developmental Stages and Tasks

Stages	Tasks
1. Setting goals	Develop desired long-term goals for the family structure based on needs of all family members
	Explore possible roles for the stepparent in relations to the stepchildren
2. Parental limit setting	Biological parent in the stepfamily in charge of setting and enforcing limits for biological child
	Stepparent sets limits in accordance with biological parents' rules
	In a family where both spouses have children, the couple will need to accept the existence of different rules for different children
3. Stepparenting bonding	Create periods of time free from limit setting for stepparent nurturing of the stepchild to allow stepparent–child bonding
4. Blending family rules	Stepfamily develops own new rules and traditions
	Negotiate regarding the stepparent parental role (begins only after the initial bonding phase completed)
	Disagreement regarding rules resolved by the biological parent
	Biological parent accommodates the stepparent regarding rules to the extent that the stepparent contributes positively to the child's development
5. Stepfamily's relations in the binuclear family	Stepparent supports the child's relationship with the same-sex parent in the other household
	Differentiate between the two binuclear households

in assessing, guiding, and evaluating the family's task accomplishments relevant to the stepfamily life cycle. The stages and tasks are shown in Table 2.10.

Comparison of Professional and Low-Income Family Life Cycle Stages

The family life cycle of low-income families may not match that of the middle-class and/or professional family as discussed previously. The clinician must consider the effects of socioeconomic status (SES), environment, race, culture, ethnicity, and spirituality in how and when a family makes its transitions within its own life cycle. Hines (1988) suggested the low-income family life cycle has three phases:

Phase 1—unattached young adult (can be younger than twelve years old) who is virtually unaccountable to any adult

Phase 2—families with children—this phase occupies most of the life span including three- and four-generational households

Phase 3—grandmother who continues to be involved in central childrearing in her senior years

In 1996, 6% of all U.S. children under 18 lived with their grandparents, whereas in 1950 this was only 3% of the population (Saluter & Lugaila, 1998). Fulmer (1989) suggested a comparison of the life-cycle stages of low-income and professional families, including factors of pregnancy, education, and time, which may be helpful when working with these families. Table 2.11 illustrates the comparison of these two types of families by age.

Adoptive Family Life Cycle

The adoption experience—the decision to adopt, the application, and final adoption—can be a very stressful, as well as joyful time. This is a time when family boundaries are expanded/extended and realigned. Reitz and Watson (1992) defined *adoption* as

A means of providing some children with security and meeting their developmental needs by legally transferring ongoing parental responsibilities from their birth parents to their adoptive parents; recognizing that in so doing we have created a new kinship network that forever links those two families together through the child, who is shared by both. (p. 11)

The new legal status of the family does not sever the emotional and psychological ties the child will have to his or her family of origin. Due to various statistical systems, the actual number of children who are adopted each year is sketchy. In 1992, 127,441 children were adopted in the United States, a slight increase from 118,000 five years earlier (Fein, 1998). Approximately 42% of those adoptions involved stepparents and relatives. The biggest increase has been in children adopted from abroad, with 13,620 being adopted in 1997— almost double that of 1990 (Fein, 1998).

Adoptive families may have additional concerns during the developmental stages. During the preschool developmental stage, the family must acknowledge the adoption as a fact of family life (Wright & Leahey, 2000). There may be times within the family when the question of permanency of the relationship will surface. It is most helpful for both the children and family to talk about this openly and in a reassuring manner. During the adolescent or launching developmental stage where there is emphasis on increasing the flexibility of family boundaries, disagreements may occur that include threats of desertion or rejection within adoptive families. In the launching stage, the young adult "adopts" the parents in a re-contracting phase (Hajal & Rosenberg, 1991). In the middle years stage when the adopted children are structuring their own families, the integration of the adoptee's biological progeny can be a developmental challenge. Although adoptive parents may be delighted with commitment to these grandchildren, the biological children may or may not find this very distressing.

Alternatively, adoptive parents may mourn the loss of biological grandchildren and the pain of genealogical discontinuity. The adoptee may have simultaneous feelings of happiness at having her or his own children while being uneasy of the unknowns in her or his own genetic heritage. Adoptive parents must adapt to these concerns as well as the personal and interpersonal stress that accompanies parenthood. Table 2.12 identifies other developmental transitional issues and stresses that may be experienced by adoptive parents.

Many agencies offer adoption in an open manner. Silverstein and Demick (1994) outlined potential benefits for those involved. For the birth parents, benefits include increased empathy for the adoptive parents, reassurance that the child is safe and loved, and a reduction of shame and guilt. Benefits for the adoptive parents include increased empathy for the birth parents, reduced stress imposed by secrecy and the unknown, and an embracing at the beginning of an affirmative acceptance of the child's cultural heritage. For the child, benefits include increased empathy for the adoptive parents, enriched connections with them, and reduced stress of disconnection while simultaneously there is increased empathy for the birth parents with a decrease in fantasy about them. With clear and consistent information, the child has an increase in control in dealing with adoptive issues. The benefits are significant when forming the new family, especially when adopting children from different cultures, ethnic groups, and races. Children are also adopted into various types of family structures: divorced, single-parent, married, remarried, gay/lesbian, and extended. Some adoptive families may have a form of open dual parentage.

Although there are many adoptions that fare well, there is an over representation of adopted children in the mental health outpatient system (Hajal & Rosenberg, 1991). They have developed the following hypotheses to explain this:

- Genetic, hereditary factors
- Deficiencies in prenatal and perinatal care
- Adverse circumstances of adoption, including multiple disruptions in early life
- Conditions in the adoptive home, including pre-existing family problems
- Temperamental differences between the adoptee and the adoptive parents/family

Table 2.11.
Comparison of Low-Income Family and Professional Family Life Cycle Stages

Age	Low-Income Families	Professional Families
12-17	First pregnancy	Prevent pregnancy
	Attempts to graduate high school	Graduates from high school
	Parent attempts strict control before pregnancy. After, relaxation of controls and continued support of mother/ infant	Parents continue support while permitting child to achieve greater independence
18-21	Second pregnancy	Prevent pregnancy
	No further education	Leaves parental household for college
	Young mother acquires adult status in parental household	Adapts to parent/child separation
22-25	Third pregnancy	Prevent pregnancy
	Marriage: leaves parental household to establish step-family	Develops professionalism in graduate school
	Maintain connection with kinship network	Separates from parents, begins living in serious relationship

26-30	Separates from husband	Prevent pregnancy
	Mother becomes head of own household within kinship network	Marriage: develops nuclear couple as separate from parents
		Intense work involvement as career begins
31-35	First grandchild	First pregnancy
	Mother becomes grandmother and cares for daughter and infant	Renew contact with parents as grandparents
		Differentiate career and childrearing roles between husband and wife

Source: From Fulmer (1989). In Carter and McGoldrick, *The changing family life cycle: A framework for family therapy* (2nd ed.). Published by Allyn and Bacon, Boston, MA. Copyright © 1989 by Pearson Education. Reprinted by permission of the publisher.

Table 2.12.
Development Issues and Stresses of Adoptive Parenthood

Developmental Issue	Stresses
No role model	Difficulty developing realistic expectations about the transition to adoptive parenthood
	Preparation for parenting tends to be based on experiences with own parents
Timing of transition role	Uncertainty about the transition to parenthood—may be anywhere from a few months to six to seven years
	Absence of usual pregnancy cues makes it difficult for others to alter perceptions and expectations of couple becoming parents
In-depth evaluation process	Proving their worthiness to be parents
	Process perceived as intrusive and anxiety-arousing
Timing of adoption placement	Extent of attachment bonds between child and biological or foster parents
Biological risk associated with adoption	Background of child—genetic, parents' behavior, prenatal/birth complications
Telling child about adoption	Makes explicit that adoptive parents are not biological parents
	Introduces image of natural parents into adoptive family system
	Threatens exclusiveness of relationship between adoptive parent and child

Source: Stanhope and Lancaster (1996).

- Fantasy system and communication regarding adoption, including parental attitudes about adoption
- Difficulties establishing a firm sense of identity during adolescence
- Greater age differences than usual between parents and adoptee

Clinicians who are dealing with adoptive families or adoptees should consider these factors when helping adoptive families or adoptees. Although all of these hypotheses may not apply to the family or adoptee, being aware of these possibilities will assist in a productive assessment and outcome.

Foster Family Life Cycle (Children in Foster Care Custody)

The number of children in foster care custody has increased substantially over the past two decades—up 60% from 1982 to nearly 480,000 children in 1995 (Barbell, 1997). Current national estimates are that more than 500,000 children are in a foster care setting (Leslie, et al., 2000). The increasing number of children in foster care reflects the increasing number of substantiated abuse and neglect reports, more entries than exists into foster care, and the impacts of poverty, prenatal drug and alcohol use, family violence, homelessness, and AIDS on at-risk families (Barbell, 1997).

"Investigations over the past 20 years have highlighted the extent and seriousness of the physical and mental health problems experienced by children entering the foster care system. Current estimates of mental health problems range from 30% to 80% with 40% to 80% of these children experiencing some chronic health problems, 43% showing growth abnormalities, and 33% having untreated health problems" (Horwitz, Owens, & Simms, 2000, p. 59).

Children who enter the foster care system come from a family system that is at risk for abuse and neglect and that has complex, rather than simple factors affecting their family functioning. Landy and Munro (1998) proposed a number of factors at the individual (child and parent), family, and community/cultural levels that "place parents 'at risk' for abusing and neglecting their children and their children at risk for compromised development" (p. 307; see Table 2.13). Dealing with up to four of these factors is manageable for some parents, but beyond this number each risk factor is more than additive and multiplies the risk dramatically. Also, if some of the more significant factors occur at the highest negative end of the spectrum, the situation can become increasingly precarious (Sameroff & Fiese, 1990).

Chu (1992) noted that survivors of severe childhood abuse often display great difficulty in functioning. These difficulties can include posttraumatic stress symptoms, dissociation, impulse control problems, and difficulties in secure attachments or relationships with their children (Herman, Perry, & van der Kolk, 1989; van der Kolk, Perry, & Herman, 1991). These parental factors, along with factors putting the family at risk for abuse and neglect, often propel the children into the foster care system, living with a foster care family often

Table 2.13.
Levels of Risk Factors for Child Abuse and Neglect

Child Level	Parent Level	Interaction Level	Family Level	Community Level
•Low birthweight	•History of abuse/neglect	•Poor use of discipline techniques	• No support	•Chaotic and violent neighborhoods
•Prematurity	•Placements in foster care	•Parent lacks sensitivity and attunement with child	•Recent life stress	•Lack of community support systems
•Biological/congenital difficulties	•History/current physical illness	•Insecure attachment of child to parent	•Inadequate income/ housing	
•Difficult temperament	•Major losses in childhood	•Parent rejects child	•Several children	
•Significant delays or learning disabilities	•Dysfunctional family of origin	•Parent considers child as a burden	•No partner	
•Failure to thrive	•Poor education, employment	•Parent lacks parenting knowledge	•Violence in the family	
•Feeding problems	•Low intellectual functioning		•Lack of support from partner/extended family	
•Lack of responsiveness	•Less than Grade 10 education		•Dysfunctional family	
•Frequent infections/ illnesses	•Single teenage motherhood		•Poor development of previous children	
	•Criminal record/activities		•Sibling abuse	
	•Failure to attach to child		•Frequent moves	
	•Abuse of previous children		•No telephone	
	•Alcohol or drug misuse			
	•Mental illness/depression			

Table 2.14.
Developmental Issues for Foster Family Formation

Steps	Developmental Issues
1. Removal from biological family	Separation and/or abandonment issues
	Dealing with loss of and fears at removal from family and possibly siblings
2. Entry into custodial care	Fears and uncertainty regarding the unknown for self and possibly siblings
	Anger and resentment at being removed form biological family
	Uncertainty, fear of legal issues related to self and family
3. Entering the foster family	Fear of the unknown
	Adjustment to new boundaries, space, time frame, family membership, authority
4. Adjustment to foster family	Realignment of relationships
	Encountering the unknown of permanent placement
	Maintaining connections to biological, extended family
	Loyalty conflicts
5. Adjustment to the unknown	Fears and anxiety over outcome of placement Integrating into new family rules and roles
6. Resolution of custody	Final resolution of family disruption Possibly having to accept permanent removal from biological family
	Anger and resentment at being removed from biological family

for an undetermined amount of time. Developmental issues for foster family formation are listed in Table 2.14. These steps and developmental issues could be used as a guide by clinicians in assessing, guiding, and evaluating the family's transition during this phase of the family life cycle.

Aging Family Life Cycle

The growing number of elderly people and their percentage in the general U.S. population has had a significant impact on the country's economy and its health and social services. By the year 2040, the United States will have more people over the age of sixty-five than under twenty years of age (U.S. Bureau of the Census, 1995). Among the elderly, the fastest, growing groups are minorities, the poor, and those aged eighty-five and over. By the year 2030, the minority population will make up 25% (up from 13% in 1995) of all ages (Harper, 1995; U.S. Bureau of the Census 1995).

The elderly population can be categorized as: sixty-five to seventy four "young–old," seventy-five to eight-four "middle–old," and eighty five and above "old–old." A distinction should be made in the family dynamics and the needs of persons in the age group eighty-five and over and the elderly who have not reached that age. There are noticeable differences between individual family members in their sixties and persons in their eighties. The younger group is relatively healthy, whereas persons in the older group are much more vulnerable, frail, and at risk for visual problems, cognitive impairment, and falls. They also have limited economic resources and community supports, and are more affected by chronic diseases and disorders of aging (Ebersole & Hess, 1994). The increasing numbers of older adults, combined with the ever increasing mobility and distance between family members' residences, are salient factors to be considered by those working with American families in the twenty-first century.

Clinicians working with older adults and their families must be able to evaluate the aging, dysfunctional family. Just as a fever is not pathogenomic for a particular infectious agent or disease yet is critical to a medical diagnosis, the complaint that "my family no longer loves me" does not reveal the specific problems within the family (Blazer, 1984). However, it does accentuate the need to assess the potential of that family to provide care and support for the older adult. Clarification of the nature of the family structure in interaction, the presence or absence of a crisis within the family, and the type and amount of support available to the older adult family member are essential in a comprehensive diagnostic family work up.

A genogram tracing behavioral patterns within the family is essential. The addition in the genogram of the details of the distribution of illnesses across a family is particularly helpful when working with older adults. A review of roles of individuals in the family and the availability of members to provide support and care to the older adult is equally important and may be facilitated by use of an ecomap. In providing care for families, it is important to remember that the family consists not only of individuals genetically related, but also those who have developed relationships and are living together as if they were related (e.g., nursing home residents, retirement community residents, older adults sharing private housing). Many older adults, especially those who have been widowed, have close relationships with friends that are virtually familial (Blazer, 1996).

Blazer described certain roles that family members fill in the family systems of older adults. These roles are useful in the evaluation and planning of both individual and family intervention. They include the following:

Facilitator: The individual in the family who resists intervention in order to maintain the stability achieved within a family, secondary to the older adult's dysfunction. They can present obstacles even though they believe they are being helpful.

Victim: The individual in a family who perceives the dysfunction of the older adult as a threat to self. The victim is usually in frequent contact with the older adult and therefore is in frequent contact with the clinician. The clinician may be criticized by the victim because of the burden of the older adult's dysfunction.

Manager: The family member who takes charge of a family during a crisis. This individual is usually calm, tends to organize and direct family activities, often from a distance.

Caregiver: The family member who nurtures the older adult. This individual may provide inexhaustible help and may suffer a severe and prolonged grief reaction if the older adult dies and the family system is unbalanced.

Escapee: The escapee is the family member who may withdraw from usual interactions within the family and who is blamed for not demonstrating concern and care for the older adult. This person usually lives a great distance from the older adult and frequently is seized with conflict at the prospect that the previously functional family has become dysfunctional secondary to health or other dysfunctional needs of the older adult.

Identified Client: This is the older person with the problem, who is perceived to be the cause of a family crisis. The identified client may suffer only minimal problems and may be content with his or her present state. Yet the older adult may provide a token, a reason, for the entire family to seek therapeutic intervention. The needs and problems of the older adult may quickly be set aside as family conflicts emerge during evaluation and ongoing treatment.

Therapeutic intervention with an aging family is a pandimensional and poly-faceted endeavor. It is complicated by the fact that traditional developmental theories such as those of Erikson and Piaget do not address, nor take into consideration, a phenomenal increase in the life span of the average individual living in the American society and culture of the twenty-first century. In her classic book, *Family Development,* Duvall (1971) made a major contribution among nurse theorists in that she actually addressed the concept of family within the scope of nursing care. Her family development theory is, however, woefully inadequate in dealing with the aging family, as its stages of family development are based on the age of the eldest child and issues relating to children leaving the nuclear family setting. Systems theories such as Bowen's Family Systems Theory developed in the mid-1970s and Martha Rogers' nursing theory, The Science of Unitary Human Beings, developed in 1970, refined in 1986, further refined in 1990, and continuously undergoing refinement to this date, provide and create more space for creative holistic assessment of and therapeutic intervention with the aging family.

Domestic Partner/Family Relationship Life Cycle

Domestic partnerships refer to lesbian, gay, and non-married heterosexual cohabitants who are engaged in an intimate relationship and are financially interdependent (Ames, 1992). In the early 1990s, U.S. Census data showed there were six cohabiting couples per 100 married heterosexual couples with 40% of these couples having children (Bumpass, Sweet, & Cherlin, 1991). As the U.S. population ages, often older adults, who are on a set income, will choose to live together as their financial constraints do not allow each to live on their own. Some individuals may choose to live in an intentional community where they may share their lives with other individuals as well as with other families.

Lesbian and gay individuals may choose to live in a variety of family forms. In the United States, common definitions of the family have been built on the concepts of law and nature, legal/common law marriage, and blood relatedness (Walsh, 1993). On the other hand, the nonbiological fictive (substitute) lesbian and gay family, which is not a legal marriage, not headed by heterosexual parents, and does not produce biological children, is often seen as nontraditional, alternate or deviant, exceptional, and marginal to what is considered the normal family. Gay and lesbian families defy cultural assumptions about the meaning of family, as well as the family defined by law and blood kinship. These are families formed from lovers, friends, biological and adopted children, blood relatives, stepchildren, ex-lovers, and families that do not necessarily share a common household.

Gay families devise a new system of kinship in which they "choose" their families (Slater, 1995), "retaining the familiar symbol and combining it with symbols of love and choice" (Laird, 1993, p. 294). There is no normative structure for the lesbian or gay family, as, like all families, they come in all shapes and sizes. Families with children may be headed by a single parent, a same-sex couple, or a multiple-parent extended family structure. Some lesbian families include biological fathers. "They are rich and poor, black and white, Jewish and Gentile, Italian and Armenian; except for the fact that one or more members are lesbian or gay, these families cross cut the same social categories as other families" (Laird, 1993, p. 295).

On the other hand, as same-sex couples choose and form families in which legal marriage, heterosexual partnering, and procreation are not the organizing metaphors, this family form offers an opportunity for re-examining and re-creating one's ideas about family and kinship.

With their relatively fluid boundaries and varied memberships, their patterns of non-hierarchical decision making, their innovative divisions of labor, and the relative weight given to friendship as well as blood relatedness, such families offer further challenge to dominant notions of family structure and functions and present an opportunity for mental health professionals to assess the limitations in current definitions of family and kinship. (Laird, 1993, p. 296)

Slater (1995) has applied the family life-cycle framework to the lesbian/gay family career. This five stage model (see Table 2.15) reflects the diversity and points of common experience among lesbian/gay families. This family life cycle, unlike Carter and McGoldrick's conception of the family life cycle, is not typically and traditionally child-centered and is not affirmed in the larger society. The conception and experience of family life over time is highly sensitive to the social and historical context in which the family exists. According to Friedman (1998), "The couple's adaptions to the challenges of previous stages become incorporated into their relationship and strengthen or diminish their capacity to confront subsequent obstacles. The layers of partner chronological development, lesbian/gay identity formation, other minority identity formation, and the stage of the life cycle intersect continually" (p. 142).

The clinician, when working with a gay family, must resist being seduced by the dominant culture into seeing these families as deviant or abnormal. Rather, it would be more helpful to be nonjudgmental and to see this family form as the emergence of a "pluralism" in family forms (Laird, 1993).

FAMILY CAREGIVING

When a family member has a health problem and becomes ill or disabled, the family can become the source of caregiving for the individual. Family members play a vital role as the primary caregivers for both the frail elderly as well as for family members who are dependent due to chronic physical and/or mental illness (Friedman, 1998). The amount and kind of care provided by family members is often a critical factor in determining whether or not an ill or disabled member remains at home or is institutionalized. Although families are often the first to want to provide care for other family members, the effects or risks on the family caregiver of providing this care to a family member must never be over looked (Wright & Leahey, 2000).

Family Kin Relationships

Mother. Although various members of the family may contribute to caregiving, the mother is most often seen in the role as health leader of the family. She is the central person responsible for caregiving, health decision making, education, and counseling within the family unit (Finley, 1989; Litman, 1974). In this role, mothers identify illness signs and symptoms, decide how this will be dealt with within the family unit, and then decide what family and/or community resources are needed to deal with the health problem. Due to this important and central role of the mother in the family, family functioning may become very disrupted if she becomes ill (Litman, 1974). Other family members, often the oldest female child, may take on some of the mother's roles within the family (Kahana, Kahana, Johnson, Hammand, & Kercher, 1994). When involving children in caregiving and care-rearing roles, families need to throughly understand a health problem and the chronicity of the problem in order to facilitate flexibility of roles within the family (Rolland, 1994a). This flexibility prevents one child from completely taking on one or several roles that are not age-appropriate.

Table 2.15.
Domestic Partners: Lesbian/Gay Family Career

Stage	Transition Process	Developmental Tasks
1. Couple formation	Partners need to differentiate when they began to show interest from when they began an actual couple relationship.	a. Building a beginning sense of themselves as a unit. b. Relaxing boundaries around themselves as they tentatively blend aspects of their lives. c. Developing trust between partners. d. Increasing self-disclosure. e. Engaging in empathic responses that encourage further risk. f. Controlling who knows about their relationships.
2. Ongoing couple-hood	Couple moves from unbridled passion to beginning of stability, combining passion and dailiness.	a. Recognizing and managing a range of differences that are becoming evident. b. Negotiating conflict. c. Developing relational security and sense of belonging.
3. Middle years	Couple's movement into a permanent or long-range commitment.	a. Diligent reworking of the rewards and disappointments within extended relational commitment. b. Creating security and continuing newness within the relationship.

4. Generativity	Couple's desire to associate themselves with and provide a sense of identity that will endure beyond their own finite existence.	a. Creating a personal legacy.
5. Couple over 60	Couple facing imposed life changes, some occurring all at once and others emerging, such as retirement, physical illness, and widowhood.	a. Partner renegotiation of interdependence and autonomy. b. Each partner working to secure some power and unique identity for self within the relationship. c. Balancing financial, physical, and emotional independence.

Source: Family Nursing: Research, Theory and Practice by Friedman, MM, ©. Reprinted by permission of Pearson Education, Inc., Upper Saddle River, NJ.

Taking on age-inappropriate roles would prevent the child from accomplishing his or her own age-appropriate development tasks.

When considering role relationships, mothers are most often the primary caregivers of chronically ill children (Shepard & Mahon, 1996). Although the mother acts as the primary care provider for the child, her husband or significant other may be providing support and affection to her. Women who are married have the advantages of having a husband who provides financial and socioeconomic support, and who helps with instrumental tasks (Dwyer & Coward, 1991; Horowitz, 1985; Stone, Cafferata, & Sangl, 1987). On the other hand, unmarried women report problems of loneliness, lack of support, and lack of instrumental caregiving help (Brody, Litvin, Kleben, & Hoffman, 1990).

Spouses and Adult Children. Spouses or adult children provide 80% to 90% of care for their elderly family members (Brody, 1985). This is due in part to the prospective payment system that has shortened hospital stays sending people home earlier and sicker. Often, an elderly husband will assume the care for his wife when she becomes ill or disabled (Richards, 1996). If adult children provide care, daughters outnumber sons as caregivers by four to one (Brody, 1990). Although parents may initially care for their disabled adult children, usually another sibling becomes the care provider when the parents can no longer provide care.

Multiple Caregiving Roles. Recently, family caregiving trends include increases in the number of caregivers with multiple caregiving responsibilities, grandchildren responsible for helping one or two older generations, and aging women without caregiver husbands due to the high divorce rates (Brody, 1995). The stresses that these situations bring to bear on a family when taking on caregiving have consequences that are seen by family members as having both positive and negative benefits. The following positive experiences of family caregiving have been identified: caregiver *reciprocation* through expressions of affection or appreciation toward the caregiver (Carruth, 1996); *help* from care-receiving mothers in return for their daughter-caregiver's help (Walker, Pratt, & Oppy, 1992); *companionship and help with physical house work* when older parents are caring for adult dependent children (Bulger, Wandersman, & Goldman, 1993); and *positive emotional impact* of combining multiple roles on employed caregivers (Neal, Chapman, Ingersoll-Dayton, & Emlen, 1993). Problems identified within the caregiving role include:

Significant caregiving problems identified by researchers include: coping with the increased need of the dependent family member caused by physical and/or mental illness; coping with disruptive behaviors . . . ; restrictions on social and leisure activities; infringement on privacy; disruption of household and work routines; conflicting multiple role demands; lack of support and assistance from other family members; disruption of family relationships and lack of sufficient assistance from human service agencies and agency professionals. (Biegel, Sales, & Schulz, 1991, p. 7)

Problems with the Elderly. In a study of caregivers of older persons, Harvath, Stewart, and Archibold (1994) found the management of behavior problems to be a more powerful predictor of role strain than the management of physical problems. In a large study of primary caregivers providing care to a spouse or parent with Alzheimer's disease or a related dementia, the following stressors were experienced: role overload, role captivity (feeling involuntarily trapped in the caregiver role), and the loss of intimate exchange because the ill family member has "become someone else" (Aneshensel, Pearlin, Mullan, Zarit, & Whitlatch, 1995). Also in this study, the caregiver's relationships with other family members, work, and other social roles were adversely affected.

Illness Factors

Biegel et al. (1991) identified patient illness characteristics associated with family caregiver strain including severity of the illness, amount of patient change from pre-existing condition, and suddenness of the onset of the illness problem. Additionally, contextual/caregiver variables that mediate the family caregiver's reaction include demographics (gender, role relationship, age, and SES), pre-existing psychological factors, relationship quality, family life stage, and social support. Female gender and role relationship (spouses and parents) are consistently associated with greater caregiving burden, whereas other variables show contradictory or more complex patterns.

Biegel et al. (1991) mentioned significant family caregiving problems identified by researchers with a family member with a mental illness. These included coping with the increased needs of the dependent family member caused by the mental illness. Caregivers of mentally ill relatives often sustain caregiver burden due to dealing with disruptive behaviors and providing instrumental and emotional assistance for their family member (Reinhard & Horwitz, 1995). Mental illness of a family member is a particularly traumatic stressor that can precipitate a family crisis or decompensation.

Caregiving for a Mentally Ill Family Member

There are many facets of family care that are involved when dealing with a mentally ill family member. For example, family members are often involved in the care of the member at the hospital and when he or she returns home (Cox, 1995). Additionally, families may have to deal with other institutions outside the family, such as schools, police, court officials, community agencies, and religious/spiritual organizations. The effects of these multiple aspects of care on families and their individual members must be assessed (Hatfield & Letley, 1993; Bulger, Wandersman, & Goldman, 1993).

There are some typical effects encountered by families with a mentally ill member that include the following (Gilliss, 1991; Griffin-Francell, 1993; Koontz, Cox, & Hasting, 1991; Reinhard, 1984; Sayles-Cross, 1993):

• denial, anger, fear, worry, sadness, resentment, frustration, grief, sense of betrayal, shame, guilt

- deprivation or loss of dreams, hopes, potential, expectations
- decline in sense of self-worth and self-esteem
- threat to security, well-being, safety, control, predictability
- loss of confidence, integrity, optimism
- financial strain from costs of treatment, medications
- decline in income due to absenteeism, unemployment
- decline in leisure and social activities
- decline in social support due to stigmatization
- threats to physical health due to emotional strain
- alterations in family interactions, shifts in roles, conflicts
- need for new/modified decision making, communication, stress management, coping strategies
- prolonged parenting or caregiving of an adult child
- interactions with numerous agency personnel (i.e., hospital, aftercare, rehabilitation, insurance, disability, vocational, police, financial)
- worry about future care of the family member as caregivers age

In addition to these effects of mental illness experienced by families, families also must learn to cope with family member's behaviors and problems. Some of the most common difficulties that families report when caregiving to their mentally ill family member are as follows (Hellwig, 1993; Reinhard, 1984):

- conflict between dependence and independence
- side effects of medication(s)
- noncompliance with medication and treatment
- bizarre behaviors and communication
- activities of daily living poor or absent
- exploitative and provocative behaviors
- lack of cooperation
- persistent avoidance behaviors
- lack of insight, denial, poor judgment
- social isolation
- suicidal ideation and attempts
- hostile, threatening, abusive behaviors
- intrusiveness

In conclusion, the family is often the source of caregiving for ill or disabled family members. Due to the changes within the family necessitated by this change in the family system, conflict and strain are often present, especially in the immediate period after the initial incapacitation of the family member

(Friedman, 1998). Families and/or family members are forced by circumstances to take on new responsibilities, often of the type not usually performed by the family or by a particular family member. Family members are often burdened with these changes and can feel worried, anxious, or guilty that they are not adequately performing their new job (Friedman, 1998). In the extreme, these added responsibilities may add to the family member's role to the extent that it seems excessively demanding and unmanageable.

Families respond to this situation in two ways. Either the family is able to be flexible enough to take on the basic and necessary tasks of the ill/disabled member or the family lacks the resources to perform the tasks of caring for the ill/disabled family member, thus certain tasks are not performed or are performed unsatisfactorily. The adequatly functioning family can adjust and be flexible to meet the demands of the situation or may call on resources outside the family for assistance. The dysfunctional family, however, is not able to adjust and many family tasks go undone or are done unsatisfactorily. Once the family has adjusted to the family member's illness/disability, a reintegration occurs that allows the family to then function in a new and different constructive manner.

FAMILY FUNCTIONS AND TASKS

Family Functions

At the same time that the family is evolving, the family group has functions to accomplish in order to maintain the family unit and to contribute to the society of which it is a part. Families perform many functions and these have changed over time. In his seminal work, *Social Structure*, the well-known sociologist George Murdock (1949) concluded that there are four functions of the nuclear family: sexual, reproductive, educational, and economic. In any society, the nuclear family may also have other functions that it performs and these may vary from society to society. However, these four functions are constant across all societies.

Hanson and Boyd (1996) identified some of the same family functions as Murdock, but include several others that Murdock indicated would occur. These six functions of the family have evolved traditionally, over time. These include:

1. Economic survival

2. Reproduction of the species

3. Providing protection

4. Transfer of religious faith (culture)

5. Education (socialization) of the young

6. Conference of status

According to Hanson and Boyd (1996), these six family functions have changed and new ones have been added. Friedman (1998) added two others: affective function (personality maintenance function) and health care function—provision and allocation of physical necessities and health care. This health care function includes the following:

- Maintenance of health-supporting physical and psychosocial home environment
- Resources for personal hygiene
- Provision for meeting spiritual needs
- Health education
- Health promotion
- Health-illness decision making
- Recognition of developmental disruptions
- Seeking health, dental, and illness care
- First aid
- Supervision of medications
- Rehabilitation care
- Involvement with community's health (Stanhope & Lancaster, 1996, p. 462)

Related to socialization of the young, siblings are both instigators of and recipients of the socialization process. Siblings contribute to each other and to the family in the followings ways:

1. Defending and protecting each other
2. Interpretation of the outside world
3. Teaching other about equity
4. Building coalitions
5. Bargaining
6. Negotiating
7. Mutually regulating each others' behavior
8. Serving as buffer for each other with their parents
9. Providing resources (i.e., money and material goods)
10. Establishing and maintaining family norms
11. Contributing to the family culture (Stanhope & Lancaster, 1996)

Aldous (1978) viewed sibling role behavior from a life-cycle perspective as identified in Table 2.16.

Table 2.16.
Life-Cycle Perspective of Sibling Role Behaviors

Sibling Age	Role Behaviors
Preschool	Handle competition for parents' attention
	Handle grievances toward each other resulting from parental differential treatment
School age	Develop an affectional sibling structure
	Engage in role making with siblings
	Function as discipline to siblings
	Develop power patterns within sibling subsystem
	Provide gender role socialization
Adolescent	Learn from each other how to relate to peer of opposite gender
	Serve as reminder to younger siblings that adolescent tasks can be mastered and provide information on content of task
	Become advisor and confidant to siblings
	Provide support and understanding that can ease parent–adolescent conflict
	Serve as mediator within family and between family and community
Adult	Maintain sibling contacts through obligatory parental contacts
	Maintain sibling bond
	Perform kin-keeping functions after death of parents
Elderly	Re-establish sibling relationship if necessary
	Provide comfort and support

Family Tasks

Duvall (1971) has described eight basic tasks of the family. Depending on the stage of family development, these tasks may be carried out differently by a family. Therefore, the clinician would need to know the stage of family development in order to assess if these tasks are being accomplished appropriately (McGoldrick et al., 1993). These tasks directly or indirectly contribute to the mental health of family members. The eight basic family tasks are:

1. Physical maintenance and safety
2. Allocation of resources—meeting family needs, costs, and apportioning materials, facilities, space, and authority

3. Division of labor

4. Socialization of family members

5. Reproduction and release of family members

6. Maintenance of order, authority, and decision making

7. Placement of members into the larger society—school, church, organizations, work, politics

8. Maintenance of motivation and morale; encouragement and affection; meeting personal and family crises; refining a philosophy of life and family loyalty through ritual

When working with families, the clinician needs to assess if the basic tasks are being accomplished for individuals, as well as for the family. Assessment of deficiencies in the accomplishment of family tasks alerts the clinician to problem areas for the family.

TRIANGLE OF FAMILY HEALTH

Clinicians need a holistic, contextual view of family problems in order to take advantage of opportunities to participate in family-level problem solving and change. The Triangle of Family Health (see Figure 2.1) provides a context to assess and understand both internal and external factors that can affect families and family change (Cox, 1999). The health of individual family members with an acute illness, such as when the mother of an infant has the flu, can

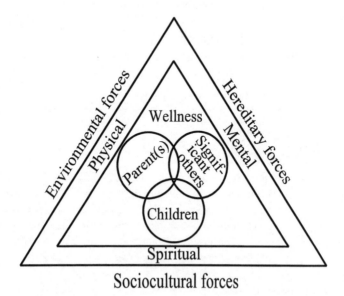

Figure 2.1. Triangle of Family Health
Source: Cox (1999).

change how a family will function temporarily, while a member with a chronic disease, such as Alzheimer's, can permanently transform family functioning. How a family deals with a family member who is an alcoholic—does the family ignore it or confront the person?—affects the individual's and the family's health.

Illness can also affect the family's subsystem (Rolland, 1994b). From these examples, it can be seen that the family affects the individual's health and the individual's health affects the family (Doherty & Campbell, 1988). When working for family change, brief, episodic family interventions are more useful due to the short time that clinicians often work with families (Cox & Davis, 1993).

Internal Factors Affecting Family Health

Research has shown that a family or marriage has effects on health (e.g., physical, psychological, and spiritual health). There is a positive relationship between marriage and physical health. Marriage appears to have a supportive and protective influence on physical health (C. Ross, Mirowsky, & Goldstein, 1990). The additional support and higher income have both been associated with better physical health. Married persons are less likely to engage in risky lifestyle behaviors and are more likely to live healthier lives (Venters, 1986). Strong and DeVault (1993) reported that husbands and wives are more likely to eat nutritiously, and are less likely to smoke or drink excessively or take risks that increase accidents. Although most relationships between marriage and health are positive, Venters (1986) found that married persons are more likely to be overweight and to exercise less.

Marriage generally improves and protects psychological health just as it does physical health (C. Ross et al., 1990). Married persons have less depression, anxiety, and other forms of psychological distress than unmarried individuals (Gore & Mangione, 1983; Gove, Hughes, & Style, 1983; Mirowsky & Ross, 1989). On the other hand, marriage has a more positive impact on men's psychological health than on women's in that men seem to benefit from emotional support and women benefit from the economic support they gain in marriage (C. Ross et al., 1990).

Children affect parenting positively and negatively. Parents with children living at home experience more psychological distress than people without children or parents whose children have left home (Kandel, Davies, & Raveis, 1985; McLanahan & Adams, 1987; C. Ross, et al., 1990; Umberson & Gove, 1989). Conversely, parents also indicate living has more meaning when children are present (Umberson & Gove, 1989). Other factors influencing psychological health are the age of the children and whether the parents are married.

When considering the family and psychological health, much research has been done on the relationship between the family and schizophrenia (Goldstein & Strachan, 1987; Lukoff, Snyer, Ventura, & Neuchterlein, 1984). Researchers have found that poor parental communication is common in these families and is present before the symptoms of schizophrenia appear (Goldstein, 1985; Karon, 1994). Although more recent research has focused on how the family and depression, alcoholism, and anorexia nervosa are related, very little has been discovered (Hanson & Boyd, 1996).

The importance of spirituality and religion in families has been confirmed by DeFrain and Stinnett (1992). They reported that of the 3,500 families they interviewed over a sixteen-year period, spiritual well-being was identified as one of the six critical qualities of strong families. This spiritual well-being was reflected by the family members' sense of optimism, hope, meaning in their lives, ability to be more patient with each other, more forgiving, and more supportive of family relationships. A shared religious core was found to be one of the fifteen health family traits by Curran (1983). A shared religious core means there is a faith in God that plays a role in the family life, a strengthened family support system that encourages nurturing and affirming relationships, and parents who pass on the faith in a positive and meaningful manner (Curran, 1985). Conversely, some aspects of religious and spiritual beliefs or values may be detrimental to families. What constitutes a family, marriage, divorce, and remarriage, contraception use, and sexuality, may be narrowly defined by a religious institution. For families not congruent with these religious values, this can be a source of stress rather than support and comfort. Although inclusion of this aspect of family life may be seen to be an invasion of privacy, it is important for clinicians to be sensitive to how these beliefs and values influence the family's health and response to illness, especially if the family is of a different cultural heritage.

External Factors Affecting Family Health

Forces outside of the family also influence family functioning and health (see Figure 2.1). Environmental factors, such as legal and family policy, can affect family functioning and health. Legal factors include legal definitions of what constitutes a family, the federal government's involvement in family issues, and local and state court decisions about family issues (Liss, 1987), such as divorce, child support, child custody, and family violence (Walker, 1992). Broadly defined (Zimmerman, 1992), *family policy* can be any policy that impacts families such as those related to housing, health, income maintenance, education, social services, or employment.

Sociocultural factors refer to families's SES and cultural heritage. A family's SES affects the family's lifestyle, members' health status and longevity, their educational and occupational opportunities, and a multitude of other life conditions (Hanson, 2001; Hanson & Boyd, 1996). Every culture possesses a system of beliefs and practices about health and illness (Helman, 1990). These beliefs and practices affect how a family deals with health maintenance, health promotion, and illness. Health beliefs explain such things as, what a symptom is, what symbolizes relief or cure, and whom you go to for help. Families in different cultures pass on, from generation to generation, ideas about what is healthy and what is not.

Western societies have different ideas about this than non-Western societies. These health beliefs are transformed into health care practices that look very different from culture to culture. What constitutes appropriate health care is bound by cultural and social class expectations (Hanson & Boyd, 1996). "Conflicts between family members about health care beliefs and practices may adversely affect family health" (p. 87). This may leave the family divided, less capable to problem solve around health problems, and less able to care for a family member with a problem.

Although culture passes on family ideas and beliefs from one generation to the next, *heredity*, through physical means such as genes, passes on biological differences from one generation to the next (Giger & Davidhizar, 1995). Body structure, skin color, other physical characteristics, enzymatic variations, and susceptibility to disease are examples of biological variations. These hereditary, biological variations are found within all racial groups and cultures, affecting the health of individuals and families. Knowing the racial predisposition to a certain disease is helpful in evaluating and diagnosing illnesses, as well as in assessing risk factors (Divan, 1989). For example, diabetes mellitus, hypertension, and systemic lupus erythematosus are found in higher incidence among certain groups. Although heredity can make a contribution to certain illnesses, it is important to remember that susceptibility to health problems may also be affected by environmental factors or a combination of environment and heredity factors (Giger & Davidhizar, 1995).

In summary, both internal and external factors affect family functioning and health. When the emotional system of the family is understood (i.e., by using Bowen's Family System Theory and Olson's Circumplex Model, along with other internal factors that affect family health), the clinician has expanded information on which to base family interventions. As the view of the family is broadened by including external factors, the clinician has a much larger systemic view to understand all forces that may be impacting the family. Within this larger systemic view lies multiple opportunities for family system change.

FAMILY STRUCTURE AND PROCESS

Families are engaged in an ongoing evolution of change in family structure and process (Hanson & Boyd, 1996). Changes in family structure and process have implications for family-centered health care delivery. The family structure and process influence, and are influenced by, the health status of individual family members and the health of the family unit. What is the answer to these questions: How do families work? How do they do what they do? What goes on in families that affects the health of its members and the health of the entire family? Understanding family structure and process assists in answering these questions as families change over time.

Family Structure

Family structure refers to the individuals who comprise the family and the connections among them: subsystem, boundaries, roles, rules, and triangles. A definition and explanation of each is found in Table 2.17. Family structure will change gradually over time as members enter and leave the family, or suddenly,

Table 2.17.
Concepts Used in Understanding the Family

<u>STRUCTURE</u>   (FIRST thing you will see in the family)

Subsystem	basic structural units of the broader family system
	Types: spousal, sibling, social network, parental, intergenerational
Boundaries	abstract dividers that define "who is in" and "who is out"/ implicit rules
	defining who participates in which system and how
	-internal and external-all families have both of these
	-classified as: closed/open/random
	-rigidity/flexibility
Roles	who plays what part in the family?
	special interactional patterns (NOT family position as mother,
	grandmother, aunt)
Rules	define boundaries and behaviors; how things are done; functions
	Types: Procedural Rules: "how to" messages; what; when; where
	Ex.: "How does your family celebrate holidays?"
	Relational Rules: expectations about how family members should treat
	each other, to include sexuality
	Ex.: equal, unequal, cooperative, competitive, hostile, affectionately
Triangles	will always be there; when stress between two people, a third brought in
	-"perverse ▲" (Jay Haley) - breached intergenerational boundaries

---

Table 2.17.
Continued

-central ▲ -always be one there [may not be pathological/dysfunctional]

-can change over time; in large families, may have 2 ▲s

When looking at central ▲ and have *triangulation*, see either:

-Parentification - child in ▲ and pulled in too close-relationship with parents given

special status/privileges/power to function as caretaker of something in the family

-Scapegoating - push child away in order to decrease tension in marital dyad -

child often is brought into therapy as the identified client - when child gets out

of ▲, parental tension increases and get one of the following: 1. Refocus ▲ on

another child; 2. Stress in parental dyad increases and see dyad in therapy;

3. Affair; 4. Physical/emotional illness

Triangles can be in the following forms:

Coalition--when two people in a triad join forces to counteract a third

Alliance--when two people get together because of a common interest

PROCESS (quality of interactional experiences; interactive components of the system parts)

Separateness/Connectedness

-emotional closeness and distance (must be felt as cannot be seen)

-separateness-allows for individuation of each member and sexual expression

-connectedness-ties family together

Enmeshment/Disengagement

-emotional level of interactive functioning of family unit

-classify system - tends to mainly operate as either one or the other (cannot be

both or part one, part the other)

(continued)

Table 2.17.
Continued

-**Enmeshed families**-diffuse internal boundaries and more closed external

boundaries. Enmeshed systems are characterized by a high degree of emotional

connectedness and reactivity between members. There is a sense of belonging

and connectedness but less of a sense of independence-hard to separate from

family.

-**Disengaged families**-strong/rigid individual boundaries and diffuse external

boundaries. Family members may function independently but lack a sense of

belonging. Only high stress levels activate the family's support system. It may be

easy to leave home (can be premature) but the individual may have little sense of

connectedness, making intimacy difficult.

Communication

-between members of the system/least important aspect

-pure process; has multidimensional meanings; must understand

meanings/codes

-how do members communicate regarding sexuality/how expressed in family

Power

-overt-covert/implicit-explicit/who is in charge?/effective executive system?

-ethnic/cultural groups look different

-look for this over intergenerational lines

Secrets (part of a system NOT a person)

-no logical explanation of secret

-not all know-two persons may know, but others may know of it but not the secret

-significance of the secret is hidden power- role is to stabilize and protect system

Table 2.17.
Continued

Myths (broader and pervasive over several generations)

-accepted by all family members; pervades the whole system

-not based on fact or reality so more difficult to identify

SPIRITUALITY

-how each family member and the family as a whole views and expresses

his/her/their relationship with a higher/divine power or superior Being

-how does the higher/divine power or superior Being act relationallly for welfare

and beneficial change for individual family members and the family as a whole

-how do individuals and the family experience a sense of inner peace

-how do family members enjoy each moment of their life and their life within the

family unit

---

through divorce or death. How families structure their lives affects the health of the family and its individual members.

Family Process

Family process refers to the ongoing interactive components between and among family members. Although families may have similar family structures, it is the interaction among family members that makes each family unique. "Family process, at least in the short term, seems to have a greater effect on the family's health than family structure and function, and in turn, to be more affected by alterations in health status" (Hanson & Boyd, 1996, p. 67). Components of family process are separateness/connectedness, enmeshment/disengagement, communication, power, secrets, and myths (see Table 2.17 for definitions).

Family Structure and Process within Its Cultural Context

Although Chapter 4 deals in detail with culture and its affect on families, the culture in which the family resides must be considered when dealing with family health and its assessment. The family's culture dictates and thus influences the family's values, attitudes, and beliefs about factors that affect the family's health and well-being. These factors include the following: "spiritu-ality, rituals [holidays, celebrations], customs, dietary habits, child-rearing practices, health, folk diseases/folk medicine, cultural healers, care of the ill family member, and the role of spiritual leader in care for an ill family member" (Swanson & Niles, 1997, p. 324; see Figure 2.1 for spirituality). If the clinician is from a culture different than the family, then the clinician will need to educate him or herself about the culture and have the family educate him or her. If the clinician is of the same culture, he or she needs to take care not to think he or she understands the family within their same culture, as the family may have had a different cultural experience. In either case, the clinician needs to let the family educate him or her in the family's subjective cultural expe-rience.

COUNSELING POINTS

- There is no one single definition of *family*
- Families look different depending on the stage of development
- Alternative family lifestyles devise a new system of kinship
- Alternative lifestyles may challenge clinicians' beliefs and biases
- Health concerns and health promotion needs change with developmental stages
- In the coming years, the aging family will be on the increase
- Family caregiving will increase as the aging family is more prominent in our society
- Families have varied, multiple means of meeting their functions and tasks
- A holistic, contextual view of the family is most helpful in dealing with families

---

3

Theories and Concepts
How to Understand Families and Health

Ruth P. Cox and Harlene Anderson

FAMILY COUNSELING AND HEALTH: A CONCEPTUAL FRAMEWORK

A conceptual framework for family counseling and health is depicted in Figure 3-1. This framework shows how family health counseling incorporates and intersects with all levels of the family and its larger context, the community and society, where the health of each system level is considered. This framework

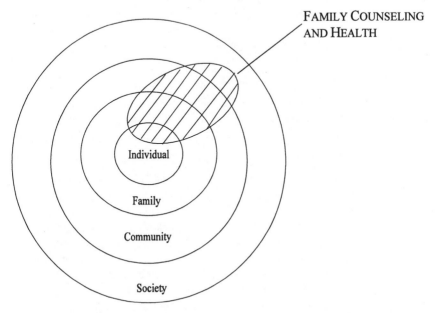

Figure 3.1. Family Counseling and Health Conceptual Framework

proposes a manner of dialoguing with families that is unique in that it purposefully incorporates all aspects of the family's health, both mental, and physical, rather than just discovering this information during treatment. This conceptual model is a metaparadigm—the *meta* referring to that which is beyond the ordinary, the most abstract understanding—the family's place and levels in its larger context of society; the term *paradigm* referring to the configuration of the concepts—the family with its individual members, their health, the family interacting with the larger context of society, and counseling. The family is understood as "both and"—it is both an entity in and of itself constituted of individual family members and it is an entity situated in the context of its larger society where counseling occurs.

FAMILY AS AN INTERACTIONAL SYSTEM
WHERE COUNSELING OCCURS

Working with "the family" can be viewed as composed of different levels of foci depending on which aspect of the family the clinician is concerned with. As discussed earlier, Doherty (1985), a family social scientist, suggested that there is a continuum for family involvement by health care provides. He suggested different severities of health problems that would necessitate involving the whole family. There has been much disagreement in the health care literature over who is viewed as the family and how it is conceptualized (Friedman, 1998), whereas in the family therapy literature the family is seen as a system where all intergenerational family members and interacting external family systems are included as the family system. Friedman suggested viewing the family on four levels when providing health care:

Level 1: The family is viewed as context to the client while the focus is on the client.

Level 2: The family is seen as a sum of the individual family members—each member is cared for individually and seen as separate rather than as an interacting unit.

Level 3: Family subsystems (parent–child; marital interactions) are the focus of care.

Level 4: The family as client where the total family is seen as an interactional system.

When considering these levels of care, family health counseling would occur at Level 4.

Wright and Leahey (1990), family nurse clinicians, suggested a perspective of the family where the concepts of *interaction, circularity*, and *reciprocity* guide the view of the family within its larger context. This view involves the interconnections between illness, family members, the family, and the larger systems characterized by holism and circular causation. Moreover, Hanson and Boyd (1996) suggested a view of the family where the family is seen as a component of society. In this view, the family is considered one subsystem, one of the many institutions within the larger system of the community—society.

FAMILY COUNSELING AND HEALTH PRACTICE:
A PRACTICE MODEL

A practice model of family counseling incorporating family health into the practice is depicted in Figure 3.2. This practice model is based on the intersection of family therapy concepts, cultural theory, and concepts of health. Family counseling and health incorporates strategies and understandings from family therapy, knowing that families are situated within their culture and its understanding of health.

OBSTACLES TO FAMILY COUNSELING
AND HEALTH PRACTICES

There are several situations that may contraindicate family assessment and counseling (Clarkin et al., 1979; Wright & Leahey, 2000). An individual may be seeking his or her own autonomy in leaving home for the first time and initially involving the family may compromise this process. Extreme schizoid

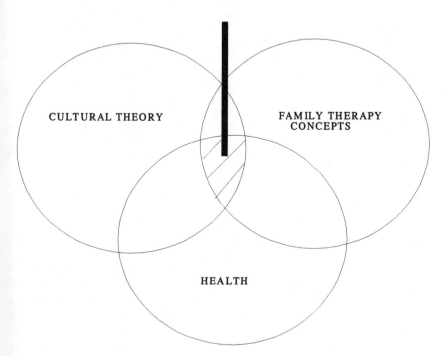

Figure 3.2. Family Counseling and Health Practice with Diverse Cultures

or paranoid pathology in an individual may not lead to a productive family interview. The individual may need resolution of repetitive intrapsychic conflicts before he or she can effectively participate in a family interview. The family may believe the interviewer is working for some institution (e.g., court, department of protective services) and therefore will not be an advocate for the family (Stanton, 1981).

Many practicing clinicians have not been exposed to family concepts in their education and thus they use an individualist approach. As well, counseling has strong ties to a focus on the individual rather than on the family. Often, counseling and health care practices regarding confidentiality have prevented the counselor from involving family members and others who have an interest in the client. Often, families have been seen as part of the problem and/or as an obstacle in providing care for the individual. At best, the family has been viewed as the context for treatment rather than as the client.

The family itself may not be convinced of the importance of family intervention (Danielson, Hamel-Bissell, & Winstead-Fry, 1993). Because most health care is individually focused and an illness, if present, is seated or isolated within an individual family member (Wright & Leahey, 2000), families may resist intervention initially not understanding the part they play in the health of the individual. In some cultures, family privacy is very important and "outsiders" are not welcomed. In some cultures, admitting that there is a "family problem" is not acceptable. For some families, getting multiple family members together at the same time can be difficult. The clinician will need to be very flexible and creative in working with families around these issues. For example, the clinician may meet with smaller subgroups of the family, sending messages home to other family members. The subgroup then may encourage other family members to attend family meetings.

System obstacles can prevent family meetings. Often, adults cannot get time off work to attend family conferences. A time that accommodates as many family members as possible can be worked out to begin with—then other members may find a way to attend. The office or clinic must be accessible to all, with enough space for wheelchairs, and must have suitable facilities. Transportation problems may prevent family members from attending meetings. Alternatives for this can be investigated so that the needs of the family are met. Insurance may not cover family meetings. If this is the case, other arrangements can be made. The office or clinic may not be convenient to all family members. Therefore, a home visit may better suit the family.

Often, the file or charting system has been oriented toward the individual and does not lend itself to focus on the whole family or on members of the family. The medical diagnostic systems used in health care have an individual focus. The *International Classification of Diseases (ICD)* and the *Diagnostic and Statistical Manual of Mental Disease (DSM-IV-TR)* have few codes that are family related. The *DSM-IV-TR* (APA, 2000a) does have some "V" code categories that are more relational focused, that is, Relational Problems, Problems Related to Abuse or Neglect when dealing with the "relational unit in which it occurs" (APA, IV, 2000a, p. 738). Presently within the U.S. health care system, these V-code diagnoses are seldom reimbursable through insurance carriers. To offset the paucity of family-focused or family-related diagnoses, the American Psychological Association (APA) does have a working group dealing with diagnoses that are family-focused. The APA does provide some information for families through its Web site, such as *Major Depression Disorder: A Patient and Family Guide* (APA, 2000b). In this guide, family therapy is one form of intervention for depression (p. 12). In the guide dealing with delirium (APA, 2000c), talking with the family is suggested during the assessment process (p. 6).

Another obstacle to the practice of counseling with families is the lack of good comprehensive family approaches and assessment models, instruments, and strategies derived from a comprehensive approach. Scholars and clinicians are developing more comprehensive models on which to base clinical practice. However, many of the present models and instruments are based on models that are narrow in scope, resulting in several instruments needing to be used to holistically assess the family. Some more recent approaches to working with the family (i.e., narrative- and solution-focused therapy), have not developed instruments for family assessment.

The Metaframeworks Perspective is not another model but rather a different approach to working with families. Breunlin, Schwartz, and Kune-Karrer (1992) conceptualize "the human condition broadly and propose a therapeutic approach that enables families to collaborate with a therapist in ameliorating the psychological suffering that arises from the human condition" (p. 23). This is done by using three building blocks, systems theory, presuppositions concerning the human condition, and six core domains. "Any theory or idea can be placed in one of these domains, as long as it is consistent with our presuppositions" (p. 23). As the authors begin with the domains and examine theories/models through the lens of the domains, the domains "can be said to transcend the models" (p. 23). Theories placed in each of the domains provide underlying patterns called *metaframeworks*. Therefore, each metaframework is a metapattern for the domain it represents. Systems theory and the presuppositions provide the underlying structure for the approach, whereas the metaframeworks (domains) provide the specifics for thinking about the human condition. Along with a flexible blueprint for therapy, which may incorporate several models, these four building blocks allow a lens to view the complexity of the human condition, without being overwhelmed by it when working with families.

HISTORICAL EVOLUTION OF FAMILY TREATMENT

The first half of the twentieth century was dominated by the psychoanalytic view that therapy should focus on the individual alone, and should not involve others or family members. This idea hindered the development of a family-level perspectives (Nichols & Everett, 1986). However, in the 1950s, three different mental health issues supported involvement of family members: couple's requests for marital counseling and therapy; parents' need for child guidance assistance; and research on schizophrenia in families.

In order to practice family-centered care, the clinician must have the "ability to think interactionally" (Wright & Leahey, 1994, p. 3), which means "to conceive (of) the individual as constantly defining and being defined by his relationships to his family and to other meaningful members of his milieu and by his insertion in the community at large" (Sluzki, 1974, p. 484). Clinicians can "think family" through a broad understanding of the family as the unit for socialization, and thorough knowledge of the combination of these two provides a framework for assessing and interviewing with families.

HOW FAMILIES MANAGE THEIR PROBLEMS

Relationship problems and conflict in families can be dealt with in several ways (Bowen, 1978; Kerr, 1981). The problems and conflict can be kept between two persons; a spouse may develop physical illness, mental illness, or have social acting-out behavior; the persons emotionally distance from each other; or a third person, usually a child, pet, or other object can be "triangled" into the conflict to reduce the tension. The person who is triangled may be seen as the "person with the problem" versus a "family problem" or the person may have disruptive behavior, such as school problems, delinquent behaviors, or health problems.

Families cope in different ways when dealing with family problems. Doornbos (1997), in his research, identified the following coping methods: assuming facilitative attitudes, relying on faith, increasing knowledge of illness, attending support groups, support of family and friends, professional assistance, and distancing from the person with the problem. Rose (1996) suggested that the stage of family development is related to the perception of stressors and identification of coping methods. When families or their members can no longer deal with conflict and the resulting relationship difficulties, they will often seek outside consultation to solve their problems.

Through a family systems perspective, the counselor accepts that the person who seeks consultation for "having a problem" provides a valuable family function as he or she becomes the reason the family can seek assistance. It is possible that the "identified client" is not ill, and when the family issues are settled, this person's functioning will return to normal as there is no need for the family's view of a "problem behavior."

In contrast, the family may have different views and/or reactions to seeking consultation for family problems (Cox, 1995). Some of these may include the following:

1. The problem lies with the "identified client" and other family members have little or no part in the problem, although they are willing to assist with treatment.

2. There is great concern that a family secret of some sort (e.g., incest) may be exposed.

3. Family members may identify the existence of a socially acceptable problem (mother's hypertension) while a more severe problem exists (e.g., spouse abuse) that the family is not willing to discuss.

4. One or both parents may exhibit concern when the client is a child and may not recognize their own part in the problem.

5. Family members may not want to be involved with the treatment of the identified client in any manner.

What ever the family's reaction to a family member's treatment, the counselor, therapist, or health care professional must be respectful and nonjudgmental in dealing with the family and the level of family members' ability to be involved in treatment.

Family Assessment Indication

A client who presents for treatment may not be living with his or her family of origin. The client may be living with a parent who has remarried several times, adoptive parents, foster parents or relatives, in a residential setting, be married or co-habitating, be a visitor in the country or an international student. The clinician must consider living arrangements when discussing with the client who is to be involved in treatment for the present problem. Although the client may not be living with his or her family of origin, present problems may be an extension of problems that existed within the family of origin. Or, individual problems may not have their origins in the family of origin, such as a recent divorce or a decision regarding becoming a parent.

Therefore, with each problem presented by a client, a judgment must be made regarding whether it should be approached within the family context. During the family assessment, the clinician must also assess for individual problems such as, suicidal, homicidal, or other risk behaviors. Situations that are common for a family assessment have been discussed previously (see the section on when to assemble the family for care).

Purpose When Working with Families

The clinician has several purposes when interviewing and working with families. These purposes begin with the initial assessment of the family and flow through to termination and referral. These purposes include the following:

1. Assessment of family characteristics—healthy and dysfunctional—in the family of origin and nuclear family

2. Prevention of dysfunction in the nuclear family

3. Intervention in normal life-cycle crises

4. Identification of health resources for troubled families

5. Provision of family education

6. Referrals to other agencies (e.g., support groups and family resources, battered women shelters, co-dependency groups, public assistance)

VIEWS OF THE FAMILY

In our understanding of families and its health, there are various ways of viewing individuals and how they are seen within the context of the family and society. In the earlier section on the family as an interactional system (Chapter 1), various views of the family were proposed:

1. Individual as the focus in the family

2. Family as the sum of individuals

3. Family subsystems

4. Family unit as the focus—both individuals and family interactions simultaneously

5. Family as a basic component of society

This chapter views the family as a basic component of society where the family interacts with other institutions in society such as health, education, religious, social, legal, and economic (Hanson & Boyd, 1996). Particular emphasis is given to the family and its interaction with health and the health care system, including the physical, mental, psychosocial, spiritual, and cultural aspects of family health. The importance of the interactions of the family with the other societal institutions also are highlighted. Clinicians dealing with the mental and psychosocial aspects of health must understand the interactions of these parts with the many other complex aspects of the individual, family, and society in order to be most helpful to the individual and family. Although the emphasis here is on the family, we should not forget that families are made up of individuals. Individuals must not be overlooked at the expense of viewing only the family—both are important. Individuals can have difficulties that are specific to themselves that may nor may not impact the family directly.

FAMILY CYCLE OF HEALTH AND ILLNESS

Every family will have phases that represent different states of family health and illness. In 1985, Doherty and McCubbin proposed the Family Health and Illness Cycle as a means of understanding the interaction within and between the family and the health care system. The family may decide to handle the health problem within the family itself, seek alternative health care, and/or seek traditional health care. The decision to seek care and what care is needed can take place in any phase of the model's cycle. With any family, the model may also look different depending on the health problem/s, family members involved, the family's spirituality, and the culturally appropriate actions to be taken. The clinician may also expect that from illness to illness, whether the same type or a different illness, what the family does and how it responds may differ with each health problem.

The Family Health and Illness Cycle proposes a view of how a family can reduce the risks of illness, manage the initial onset of illness, and adapt to illness through a temporal cycle. The model's six phases and a description of each phase are listed in Table 3.1.

In 1993, Danielson et al. synthesized the work of Doherty and McCubbin (1985) and of Coe's (1970), Stages of the Illness Experience, to establish an expanded model of health and illness relevant to the family. The eight phases of the Family Cycle of Health and Illness Model, the coping tasks, and a description of each phase are listed in Table 3.2.

Although not always possible, it is best for the family to accomplish the coping tasks for each phase during the phase of the cycle. Although the model is presented in sequential order and is often illustrated in a sequential, cyclical

Table 3.1.
Six Phases of Family Health and Illness Cycle Model

Phase	Description
1. Family health promotion and risk reduction	Emphasis on environmental, psychosocial, and interpersonal factors (beliefs and activities) that promote family health and reduce risks
2. Family vulnerability and illness onset	Susceptibility to illness or relapse of chronic illness
3. Family illness appraisal	Meaning families give to the individual's symptoms and whether the family is amenable to intervention
4. Family acute response	Response period of family immediately following the diagnosis of illness—crisis period with disorganization
5. Family adaption to illness	Role of the family in facilitating recovery or adaptation of the individual member to illness while nurturing other family members and maintaining family functions
6. Family and health care system	Decision to seek help within the family or outside the family including traditional and nontraditional treatment modalities

Table 3.2.
Eight Phases of Family Cycle of Health and Illness Model

Phase	Coping Tasks	Description
1. Family and family member health	Participate in health-promoting behaviors Participate in risk-reduction behaviors	Family members are in a state of well-being Family lifestyle of wellness behaviors
2. Family vulnerability and symptom experience	Awareness of symptoms indicating possible illness Application of folk medicine or self-medicine	Begins when family aware of symptoms of possible illness Offering of folk medicine Illness of member affects family unit Increased vulnerability to stress and illness Crisis when coping tasks not completed by either family or individual
3. Sick role and family appraisal	Acceptance of sick role by family and ill member Formation of family appraisal of and response to the situation Adjustment/adaptation of family to the sick role	Family member assumes sick role and relinquishes other roles as family begins to "experience the illness" Appraisal begins in this phase and changes as the cycle progresses Family, ill member, and support systems collaborate regarding the meaning of the illness and how it is handled

Phase	Tasks	Description
4. Medical contact—diagnosis	Establishment of relationship with health team	Health team involves family in the diagnostic process
	Gathering information about illness	Family consensus crucial to making necessary adjustments
	Acceptance of diagnosis	Cooperative relationships lessen family's struggle in this phase
5. Illness career and family adjustment/adaptation	Acceptance of treatment plan	Family finds new patterns that work as relationships change
	Family reorganization and role changes	Family exerts influence in fostering compliance with the treatment plan
	Maintain positive relationship with health care professionals	Families are consulted when making treatment plan so that the health care team can implement plan
		If crisis occurs, family may further adjust or adopt new patterns and roles
6. Recovery and rehabilitation	Relinquishment of sick role	Can occur after Phase 3 or 5
	Establishment of and adjustment to a new definition of "normal" or re-establishment of old family system	Family may keep new roles or may re-establish old patterns
		Family gives up sick-role behaviors and returns to "normal"
	Re-entering of Phase 1: Health	Recovery takes three forms: *complete* with return to "normal"; *partial* with inability to return to total sense of well-being; *disability* with recovery but not return to "normal"

(continued)

Table 3.2.
Continued

Phase	Coping Tasks	Description
7. Chronic adjustment/ adaption	Re-establishment of new definitions of normal as illness requires:	Constant adjustment as illness or family situation changes
	Learn new regimes, skills, roles	Chronic illness can assault the family or cause increased closeness
	Maintain a sense of control	
	Adjustment/adaption to altered social relationships and stigma of disability	Disabled member and family learn to adjust to new social situation
	Maintenance of positive relationship with care professional	Family must manage constantly fluctuating disabilities, shattered expectations, and chronic sorrow
	Completion of the grieving process R/T losses incurred and anticipated	Family needs clear information from health care professionals
8. Death and family reorganization	Working through the grief process	Family accomplishes family mourning tasks
	Reorganization of the family to fill vacant roles left by the deceased	Readjustment to fill vacant family roles and roles within the community and in organizations
	Realignment of extrafamilial roles	

order, the actual process for the family does not necessarily follow an exact order. "More often, the nature of the illness or the family's reaction to the illness determines the order" (Danielson et al., 1993, p. 73). For instance, a child with a broken leg can go directly from Phase 1-Health to Phase 4-Medical contact—Diagnosis. An allergic reaction to poison ivy starts with Phase 1-Health, goes to Phase 3-Sick role and appraisal, ending with Phase 6-Recovery and rehabilitation. In this instance, medical contact is never necessary and the matter is handled by the family without seeking outside assistance. It may be that folk medicine is used as advice is sought within the family system.

When a family member dies, the family's experience with illness does not end. This can launch the family into reorganization with a subsequent return to Phase 1-Health or send the family spiraling in a family stress response leading to illness, thus returning the family to the illness part of the cycle. When several family members die simultaneously or all family members die leaving one lone surviver, family roles may be undertaken by persons outside the family unit.

This model illustrates the impact that health and illness stressors can have on a family system. The clinician can use the model as a lens through which to understand how the family is managing their health and illness. As a family will make many moves around—forward and backward—through the cycle, the clinician can assist the family with their response to accomplish the coping tasks of each phase as "illness is associated with measurable social, psychological, and sometimes physical challenges for families" (Danielson et al., 1993, p. 91). Moreover, the individual's ability to cope with illness is directly related to the functional capacity of the "collective family system to manage the circumstances either positively or negatively. In this way the family serves either to enable or hinder family members as they attempt to cope with the demands of illness" (p. 91).

Illness also can affect subsystems within the family unit. For example, illness will have an impact on the relationship of the primary couple within the family (Rolland, 1994b). Illness or disability can affect the couple's intimacy and communication, either for growth or deterioration. "A number of dysfunctional structural and emotional skews are inevitable" (p. 327). These include skews related to whose problem it is, boundary issues, patient–caregiver roles, togetherness–separateness, psychosocial recovery, cognitive impairment, gender, sexuality, belief system, and life cycle.

During assessment, clinicians may want to meet with the couple both together and individually due to "patterns of secrecy and mutual protection" that often exist (p. 345). Having both individual and couple views will provide clinicians a broader understanding of the family system. A normative preventive framework that addresses the special difficulties for couples can counteract dysfunctional relationship patterns thus enhancing opportunities for increased intimacy. Addressing the skews identified here can promote a couple's resiliency by widening the range of what can be discussed or handled in the face of loss.

When working with gay, lesbian, and transsexual couples, clinicians must be aware that the couple must deal with issues related to social stigma along with the same issues that heterosexual couples face (Rolland, 1994b). Dealing with an illness may force a hidden or extremely private relationship into public for the first time, at a moment of great vulnerability. If the couple is facing a highly stigmatized disorder like AIDS, associated by society with a "deviant" lifestyle, the intensity of this experience is magnified tremendously (Landau-Stanton, 1993). A gay couple may present an intimacy that is feared by many in society and health professionals may experience discomfort in dealing with the couple. Clinicians, to be most helpful to couples, need to confront their personal prejudice and assist their clients in dealing with prejudice in others whom they encounter during the illness. Couples may need assistance when encountering their families of origin for the first time. Often a bitter family may want to restrict partner caregiving or attendance of a funeral or memorial service. As there is a variance in the legal status of gay and lesbian relationships, clinicians need to address disenfranchisement and exclusion from family leave policies and survivor benefits, lack of legal rights for visitation, and lack of legal rights for child visitation of the partner who dies (Laird, 1993).

When dealing with chronic illness, healthy coping is often dependent on the family's capacity to find or create meaning for their illness experience (Seaburn, 2001). There is often a spiritual or religious nature involved in this process. Inquiring about the family's and individual's spiritual beliefs or religious practices is an important way for clinicians to understand family identity, coping style, and orientation to life itself. Clinicians may want to involve clergy or other spiritual guides in the treatment process as they are invaluable resources for the family. Clinicians can ask questions of the family regarding the spiritual or religious nature of their family (see Chapter 5 for the types of questions that can be asked).

FAMILY PROBLEM SOLVING

When dealing with health and illness within the family, problem solving becomes a process involving various family members and is considered an aspect of overall family functioning (Bray, 1995; Fisher, 1976; Grotevant, 1989). Family-level problem solving can be defined as "the process of problem identification, solution development, and solution application by a subset of family members or the family as a unit" (Cox & Davis, 1999). Good problem-solving skills are necessary for families to resolve difficulties and manage change effectively, whether deciding on health promotion activities or dealing with an illness.

The Construct of Family Problem Solving

Tallman (1970), who made one of the earliest references to family problem solving, proposed that families who are successful problem-solvers have the following characteristics:

- Open channels of communication, such that different members can participate in problem solving at different points in the family life cycle
- Consensus among members about mutual goals and the roles of various members in the problem-solving process
- Sufficient ability among family members to discuss conflicting ideas without familial roles impeding this process
- Sufficient centralization of authority such that problem-solving efforts can be coordinated

Blechman and McEnroe (1985) proposed that families who effectively solve problems will share cues with each other during problem solving, deliberate longer, approach joint decisionmaking more carefully, use more varied strategies during a problem-solving task, and take sufficient time in problem solving in order to reach a mutually satisfactory agreement.

Epstein, Bishop, and Baldwin (1982) suggested that highly functional families are able to resolve most of their problems, whereas less functional families do not deal effectively with at least some of their problems. These authors suggested that family problem solving has seven sequential steps necessary to solve problems:

Step 1: Identify the problem.

Step 2: Communicate with those involved.

Step 3: Find alternative solutions.

Step 4: Choose a new solution.

Step 5: Implement the new solution.

Step 6: Observe the outcome of the new solution.

Step 7: Evaluate the effectiveness of the new solution.

Situational factors can affect family problem solving. For example, the nature of the health problem influences the nature and scope of problem solving as noted by Danielson et al. (1993). McCullough, Wilson, Teasdale, Kolpakchi, and Skelly (1993, p. 324) noted that acute health problems are typically well-defined issues in which family members focus on what is in the "best" interest of the (designated) client to make their decisions. In contrast, problem solving around long-term (chronic) health care problems usually requires a series of decisions over time around a constantly changing family life situation. Problem solving around health problems also is influenced by the characteristics of family members. For example, Bata and Power (1995) noted that problem solving by families with an aged member requires balancing autonomy and paternalism when identifying issues and making decisions for the older member.

Throughout the family life cycle, problem solving occurs continuously and is triggered by changes in the family, such as life situations, health status, membership, and resources. When health crises arise, families must solve problems quickly and effectively. Some families may make decisions about health-related problems as a function of well-defined family values and beliefs. Others may depend more on long-standing intrafamilial dynamics or hierarchical relationships to provide problem-solving direction. Still other families may use the counsel of health professionals for making decisions around their health problems, particularly if it is a serious or chronic problem within the family. Examples of clinical situations where family-level problem solving is important are shown in Table 3.3 (Cox & Davis, 1993).

Reliable and valid approaches for measuring family-level problem solving are necessary if clinicians and researchers are to identify and describe problem solving in both healthy and ill families, correlate family problem solving with other health and illness variables, and monitor changes in family functioning

Table 3.3.
Clinical Situations Requiring Family-Level Problem Solving

Family Situation	Family-Level Problem-Solving Issues
Health promotion	Alterations in diet, exercise, stress management practices
Pregnancy and childbirth	Role changes
	Development of parenting skills
Acute life-threatening illness	Role changes
	Development of crisis-coping skills
	Rehabilitation tasks
Progressive, chronic illness	Role changes
	Management of disability
	Acquisition of necessary self-care skills
	Adaption to functional loss
Substance abuse/ addition	Role changes
	Alterations in family dynamics
	Compliance with treatment process
Terminal illness	Adjustment to impending losses
	Management of grief and grieving
	Role changes

as an outcome of selected interventions (Cox & Davis, 1999). There are several family functioning instruments frequently cited in the clinical and research literature for measuring family problem solving. A search of the methodological literature on family problem solving yielded thirteen published family-observational or self-report measures in which family problem solving was an item, scale, or total measure. Table 3.4 provides the psychometric properties for each of these instruments (Cox & Davis, 1999).

The strengths and limitations of these instruments must be considered by clinicians and investigators who work with families in problem solving around health and illness issues. Choices from among existing family problem-solving measures also should be influenced by the intended use of the data to be collected (clinical decision making or research), the anticipated family respondent(s) and/ or clinicians who will provide those data, and the existence of rigorous and replicable procedures for administering the measure, as well as the documented psychometric performance properties of the measure. When using these instruments, clinicians need to keep in mind "cultural differences in motivation (not all minority test-takers are motivated to perform well in ability and aptitude tests), English language proficiency, and task-relevant test-taking behaviors" (Pope-Davis & Coleman, 1997, p. 18).

Interventive Questions for Family Problem Solving

For all types of family interviews, clinicians usually pose four major types of questions (linear, circular, strategic, and reflexive; Tomm, 1987, 1988; Tomm & Lannamann, 1988). Samples of each type of interview question are listed in Table 3.5. Clinicians frequently emphasize certain types of questions for the various aspects of care (Cox & Davis, 1993). For example, in collecting information concerning the main problem, many clinicians use primarily linear questions to gather information. To initiate health teaching, clinicians may use strategic questions and statements to discuss desirable health behavior changes. At times, clinicians may encounter an individual client's family members who are not known to the clinician, who may only be intermittently involved in the treatment, or who are not in agreement with the treatment process. When family-level problem solving is the goal of treatment, circular and reflexive questions may be the most useful to initiate family-level thinking about problems (Tomm & Lannamann, 1988). These circular and reflexive type questions also lead to a higher level of therapeutic alliance between the clinician and family when solving family problems (Dozier, Hicks, Cornille, & Peterson, 1998; Ryan & Carr, 2001). These approaches can be used in a variety of health promotion and prevention situations, as well as for family-focused management of crisis and/or chronic illness. Table 3.6 compares the four types of interventive questions related to the desired outcome for the family, for example, when the family is dealing with a critical illness in the family. Table 3.7

Table 3.4.
Commonly Used Family Problem-Solving Measures

Measures Model - Constructs (Authors)	Type and Use Scalar Anchors Scoring	Family Functioning Scales	Psychometric Characteristics Measurement Level	⊕ Advantages ⊖Disadvantages
McMaster Family Assessment Devise, Version 3 (Corcoran & Fisher, 1987) McMaster Model of Family Functioning Constructs-7: -Problemsolving -Roles -Communication -Affective responsiveness -Affective involvement -Behavior control -General functioning (Epstein, Baldwin, & Bishop, 1983)	Self-report - 60 items Use - clinical Scalar anchors: 4-pt. Likert-like scale, 1=strongly agree, 4=strongly disagree Score range: 1(healthy) - 4 (unhealthy) for each scale Lower score=healthier functioning	7 Scales: 1 scale for each construct	Reliability internal consistency test/retest Validity predictive concurrent construct Measurement Level -family	⊕ Differentiating healthy from unhealthy family Items clearly written, comprehensible, and unidimensional in focus Easy administration Scoring sheets and keys available making scoring easy with item indication for each subscale ⊖ Normative data limited No manual

McMaster Clinical Rating Scale (Grotevant & Carlson, 1989) McMaster Model of Family Functioning Constructs-7: -Problemsolving -Roles -Communication -Affective responsiveness -Affective Involvement -Behavior control -General functioning (Epstein et al., 1982)	Observational during clinical interview Use - clinical Scalar Anchors: 7 pt. Likert-like scale, 1=severely disturbed functioning, 7=superior functioning Score range: 1 - 7 on each scale Higher score=5 - 7 healthy functioning Lower score=1 - 4 on any scale indicates need for clinical assistance	7 Scales: 1 scale for each construct	Reliability interrater Validity criterion-related- moderate to low concurrent Measurement Level -family	⊕Identification of families in need of professional help with specific target areas Scale dimensions - well-defined anchor points Interview leading to standardization (Structured Interview of Family Functioning; Miller et al., 1994) ⊖Lack of normative data Rater training not specified

(continued)

Table 3.4.
Continued

Self-Report Family Inventory	Self-report - 36 items	6 Scales + Total	Reliability	⊕Can be used with Clinical Rating Scale
(Beavers & Hampson, 1990)	Use - clinical	Score:	internal consistency	to provide "insider" and "outsider"
		Family conflict	test/retest (30 and	perspectives of family functioning
Beavers-Timberlawn Model of	Scalar Anchors;	Family	90 days)	
Family Competence	5 pt. Likert-like scale, items	communication	Validity	Items easy to understand, respond to, and
Constructs-6:	1-34, 1=Fits our family very	Family cohesion	criterion-related	administer
-Family structure	well, 5=Does not fit our	Directive	concurrent	
-Mythology	family	leadership		Norms and manual available
-Goal-directed negotiation	Item 35, 1=family function	Family health	Measurement Level	
-Members' autonomy	well together, 5=family does	Expressiveness	-family	Children as young as 10 yrs. can
-Nature of family	not function well together			complete
-Expression	Item 36, 1=no one is	Total score		
	independent, etc., 5=family			⊖Items overlap across some scales
(Beavers & Hampson, 1990)	members usually go their			
	own way, etc.			
	Score range: 1 - 5 per scale			
	Lower score=more			
	competent family			

92

Family Awareness Scale (Corcoran & Fisher, 1987) Beavers-Timberlawn Model of Family Competence Constructs-6: -Family structure -Mythology -Goal-directed negotiation -Members' autonomy -Nature of family -Expression (Green, Kolevzon, & Vosler, 1985)	Self-report - 14 items Use - clinical Scalar Anchors: Likert-like scale- 5 pt. scale-items 1 and 2 9 pt. scale-items 3-14 - (1= very difficult; very clear; always 9= very easy; not clear; never) Score range: 14-118 Higher score=greater family competence	1 Scale: re: family competence	Reliability internal consistency Validity concurrent Measurement Level -family	⊕Identifies optimally functioning families from less competent families Can be used with all family members who can understand questions ⊖Few psychometric data available No reported normative data

(continued)

93

Table 3.4.
Continued

Clinical Rating Scale – Beavers Interactional Competence Scale (Beavers, Hampson, & Hulgus, 1990)	Observations on 10-15 min. of videotaped family interaction Use - clinical	12 Construct Scales: 1 for each construct except Invasiveness, which is a present/ absent check list	Reliability interrater Validity criterion convergent	⊕Quantitative index of family health/pathology To be used with the Centripetal/ Centrifugal Family Style Scale Scales are consistent with theoretical framework
Beavers-Timberlawn Model Constructs-13 + Global : -Overt power -Parental coalitions -Closeness -Mythology -Goal-directed negotiation	Scalar Anchors: 5 pt. Likert-like scale with 9 anchor pts. by half-pt. gradations; anchor descriptors vary	1 Global Scale	Measurement Level -family	Videotaping allows raters to replay tapes, increasing rater reliability
-Clarity of expression -Responsibility -Invasiveness -Permeability	Score range: 1 -10 for each scale			⊖Considerable training necessary with mastery of family systems theory
-Range of feelings -Mood and Tone -Unresolved conflict -Empathy -Global Health/Competence (Beavers, Hampson, & Hulgus, 1990)	Lower score= healthiest			Scales have unclear continuum Norms not available Anchor points are poorly defined on some scales

94

		2 Construct	Reliability	
Family Adaptability and Cohesion Evaluation Scale-III (Olson, Portner, & Lavee, 1985)	Self- report - 20 items Use - clinical and research	Scales: Cohesion Adaptability	Reliability internal consistency test/retest (4 wk.)	⊕Classifies families according to 16 types of functioning Measures Perceived and Ideal family functioning
Circumplex Model of Marital and Family Systems	Scalar Anchors: 5 pt. Likert-like scale, 1=almost never, 5=almost always		Validity construct	Extensive manual Clinical cut-off scores Easy administration and scoring Suitable for 9 yr. olds
Constructs -2: -Cohesion Emotional bonding Supportiveness Family boundaries Time and friends Interests and recreation -Adaptability Leadership; Negotiation Discipline; Roles and rules (Olson et al., 1985)	Score range: 10 -50 (Olson & Tiesel, 1991) Higher cohesion=very connected family Higher adaptability=very flexible family (Olson & Tiesel, 1991)		Measurement Level -family -couples without children in the home	⊖Communication is not evaluated Dimensions of constructs are not identifiable For healthy families, family functioning and scores are linearly related (Olson & Tiesel, 1991)

(continued)

Table 3.4.
Continued

Clinical Rating Scale (Olson, 1990)	Semi-structured interview	3 Construct Scales:	Reliability	⊕Allows clinician to make global rating of marital and family systems
Circumplex Model of Marital and Family Systems	Use - clinical	1 scale for each construct	interrater	Based on the above, the family is placed on the Circumplex Model grid, giving the clinician some direction for intervention
Constructs-3:	Scalar Anchors:		Validity	Does have a specific scale for problem negotiation
-Cohesion	Likert-like scale-		None available	
Emotional bonding	Cohesion -1=disengaged			
	8=enmeshed			Brief manual available
Family involvement; Marital and parent-child relationship;	Adaptability -1=rigid		Measurement Level	Communication is evaluated
Internal/external boundaries	8=chaotic		-family	No training necessary
-Adaptability	Communication -1=low		-couple	
	6=high			
Leadership; Discipline and negotiation; Roles and Rules	Global Score range: 1 - 8;			⊖No specific format is prescribed for the semi-structured interview
-Communication	Communication rated: 1 - 6			No standardization or norms
Listener and speaker skills	Middle score= best for			Communication rating is not utilized when placing family on grid
Self-disclosure	Cohesion and Adaptability			
Clarity	Higher score= best for			Inattention to rating scale issues
Continuity/tracking	Communication			
Respect and regard				
(Olson, 1990)				

Family Crisis Oriented Personal Evaluation Scales (McCubbin, Olson, & Larsen, 1981)	Self-report - 30 items	5 Construct	Reliability	⊕Purpose: to record problem-solving
	Use - clinical and research	Scales: 1 for each construct	internal consistency	attitudes and behaviors with which
purpose: identify problem-solving and behavioral strategies used by families			test/retest (4 wk.)	families respond to problems
	Scalar Anchors:	1 Total score	Validity	Provides information on which to base
	5 pt. Likert-like scale:		construct	interventions
	1=strongly disagree			Manual available
	5=strongly agree			Easy administration, scoring, clearly
Family stress theory			Measurement Level	written, and reading level simple
	Score range: total - 145-170		-family	Norms available for adults and
Constructs-5:	scales vary due to number			adolescents by gender
-Acquiring social support	of items in each scale			Norms available for families and single
-Reframing	Higher scores=more			families, African American, and
-Seeking spiritual support	successful adaptation to			Caucasian
-Mobilizing family to acquire and accept help	stressful situations			⊖Because all items are positively keyed,
-Passive appraisal				instrument vulnerable to response and
				social desirability bias
(McCubbin et al., 1981)				Variation in interpretation of anchor points
				may occur as each family member may
				view the problem differently

(continued)

Table 3.4.
Continued

Family Functioning Index (Grotevant & Carlson, 1989)	Self-report or interview - 15 items	Scale: 1 Total scale score re: desirable functioning	Reliability test/retest (6 wk. and 5 yr. for total score)	⊕Screening to examine relationship between family functioning and children's (with chronic illness) psychological adjustment who are in need of further evaluation
Sociological family role theory	Use - clinical and research			
	Scalar Anchors:		Validity	Short and reading level appropriate
Constructs-6:	5 pt. Likert-like score, 0 - 4, except two items for marital satisfaction that have a possible combined score of		construct	Good for single-parent families due to number of items for marital adjustment
-Marital satisfaction				
-Frequency of disagreement				
-Happiness	11		Measurement Level	⊖No manual
-Communication			-family	No uniform response format
-Weekends together	Score range: 0 - 35			Confusing scoring instructions
-Problemsolving				No normative data
	Higher score= more desirable functioning			"Index" to indicate families requiring further attention, not a scale to measure them precisely
(Pless & Satterwhite, 1973)				

Family APGAR (Smilkstein, 1978)	Self-report - 5 items	1 Scale re: functional family status	Reliability internal consistency	⊕Provides a database reflecting client's view of five functional states of his or her family
Family and sociological literature	Use - clinical and research		Validity concurrent content construct	Designed for use with traditional and nontraditional families
Constructs-5:	Scalar Anchors: 3 pt. Likert-like scale, 2=almost always 0=hardly ever			Easy to administer and score
-Adaptation				
-Partnership (decision making)	Score range: 0 - 10		Measurement Level -family	Can be used with children ages 8 and over
-Growth	High score= 7-10=highly functional			
-Affection	Mid-range= 4-6=moderately dysfunctional			⊖Only one item to measure each concept
-Resolve	Low score= 0-3=severely dysfunctional			
(Smilkstein, 1978)				

(continued)

Table 3.4.
Continued

Family Problem Solving	Self report - 10 items	2 Construct scales;	Reliability	⊕Developed to measure positive and
Communication	Use - research	1 for each	internal consistency	negative patterns in family problem
(McCubbin, McCubbin, &		construct	test/retest	solving and resiliency
Thompson, 1988)	Scalar anchors: 4 pt. Likert-			
	like scale, 0=false 3=true	1 Total score	Validity	Manual available
Resiliency Model of Family			concurrent	
Adjustment and Adaptation	Score range: each scale-0 -		content	Easy to administer and score
	15		construct	
Constructs-2:	Total scale: 0 - 30			Norms and comparative data available for
-Affirming communication			Measurement Level	several different populations
-Incendiary communication	Affirming score: higher		-family	
	score = positive attribute			⊖In early stages of development
(McCubbin et al., 1988)	Incendiary score: higher			Limited psychometric properties due to
	score = negative attribute			limited use

100

			Reliability	⊕Developed to assess an individual's perceptions of problem-solving behaviors and attitudes, not actual problem-solving skills
The Problem Solving Inventory (Kramer & Conoley, 1992)	Self report - 35 items 3 are research items leaving 32 items from which measures are derived	3 Construct scales: 1 for each construct	internal consistency test/retest (2wks-.83-.89; 3wks-.77-.81)	Manual clearly written and easy to use
				Short, easy to administer and score
Family literature	Use - research Scalar anchors: 6 pt.	1 Total score= general problem-solving ability	Validity concurrent discriminent content construct	Equal number of positively and negatively worded items to prevent response bias
Constructs-3: -Problem-solving confidence -Approach-Avoidance style -Personal control	Likert-like scale, 1=strongly agree 6=strongly disagree Score range: Problem-solving confidence-11-66			Individual or group administration
				⊖In early stages of development- overlap of scales measuring similar constructs
(Heppner, Cook, Strozier, & Heppner, 1991)	Approach-avoidance style-16-96 Personal control-5-30 Total scale: 32 - 192		Measurement Level -individual focus, but can be used in a family setting	Limited psychometric properties due to lack of representative normative data with the newest version of the test
				Lack of machine-scoring with test forms
	Low score= positive appraisal of problem-solving ability			Small print size in the test form
				Reading level may be too high for some adults
				Not for use with those under 16 yrs. old

(continued)

Table 3.4.
Continued

Interaction Behavior Code (Touliatos, Perlmutter, & Straus, 1990)	Observations on 10 min. of tape-recorded interactions of adolescent and parent(s)	8 Construct scales; 1 for each construct	Reliability interrater- .82-.93	⊕Developed to assess positive and negative interactions between adolescents and their parents
	Use - clinical		Validity	
Family literature	Scalar anchors: On 22 positive/ negative behaviors--1=presence;		none available	Scores discriminate between distressed and nondistressed families
Constructs-8:	0=absence			
-Positive parent behavior	Scoring: Presence of nine types of interactions--3 pt.		Measurement Level	Short, easy to administer and score
-Positive adolescent behavior			-mother/child	
-Negative parent behavior	Likert-like scale, 0=no, .5=a little, 1=a lot		-father/child	Dyad or family administration
-Negative adolescent behavior			-family (both parents and child)	
-Resolution				
-Insult	Two constructs rated on a 4 pt. scale			⊖Limited psychometric properties due to limited use
-Friendliness				
-Problemsolving	Two constructs rated on a 5 pt. scale			
	Scores computed on average ratings by 4 independent raters			
(Prinz & Kent, 1978)				

Source: Cox and Davis (1999). *Journal of Family Nursing* (5/3), 335–349, copyright © 2002 by Sage Publications, Inc. Reprinted

Table 3.5.
Four Types of Interview Questions

Type of Question	Intent of Question	Sample Questions/Statements
Linear	▪ Fact/content investigation	"How are you doing with your diet changes?"
	▪ Defining a problem	"What's the major problem that brought you all in to see me today?"
	▪ Explaining a problem	"Are you having any problems with your medication?"
Strategic	▪ Directly influencing the client system	"Why is it you are not talking about your concerns?"
	▪ Correcting "wrong" ideas, beliefs, actions	"If you all would talk with your daughter when she gets upset instead of sending her to her room, she probably would not get upset so often."
	▪ Directing client attention to specific areas	"Can't you stop arguing with your daughter about the need for changes in her children?"
Circular	▪ Pattern exploration	"How do you see that your getting upset about the grandchildren's religious practices are related to your daughter not talking with you?"
	▪ Finding connection in the client's ideas, feelings, contexts	"When your daughter gets upset about the children, who in the family comforts her?"
Reflexive	▪ Indirectly influencing the client system	"If you were to think about this differently, what other actions might you take to solve the problem?"
	▪ Facilitative of client system choices	"Do you think it would be better to talk first with your parents about your concerns, or with your husband?"

Source: Adapted from Tomm (1988).

gives example intervention questions as they are used to assist families in working through the seven family-level problem-solving steps.

Family-level problem-solving sessions can be initiated in various ways. Most clinicians initially will encounter an individual with a health problem (Cox & Davis, 1993). When client and clinician agree that problem solving needs to be accomplished at the family level, the family is invited in for the sessions. Using interventive questions can be useful to help families develop consensus about the personal meanings of specific health phenomena and the collective actions they might initiate to manage them. At the first family session, the clinician elicits from each family member his or her understanding of the problem. The clinician then meets with the family as a whole to establish possible solutions for the problem through their mutual problem solving. The clinician and

Table 3.6.
Comparison of Four Types of Intervention Questions

Type of Question	Intent	Purpose	Desired Family Outcome
Linear	Investigative	Identify the family's problem Assess family level of understanding and reaction to situation (i.e., critical care situation)	Identification of family's level of understanding and reactions to critical care situation
Strategic	Informative	Assist family in acquiring new information about event (i.e., critical care situation)	Assimilation of new information about critical care situation
Circular	Exploratory	Explore with family members their past successful coping patterns as possible means for managing current experience	Identification of past and present coping mechanisms for dealing with stressful situations
Reflexive	Facilitative	Facilitate family-level problemsolving in current situation	Consideration of new coping patterns as solutions for current critical care situation

Source: Davis and Cox (1995). Using interventive questions to empower family decision making. *Dimensions of Critical Care Nursing, 14*(1), 50. Lippincott Williams and Wilkins ©.

family would then set a date for another session at one or more months after the last session to assess the effectiveness of the solution. Subsequent sessions might be needed to monitor the problem.

THEORIES AND MODELS FOR FAMILY CARE

A theory is a general principle that can anticipate and make sense of a large and diverse range of events (Nye, 1979). Clinicians working with clients and their families will encounter many different ideas about the components of the family's problem. Theories guide professionals in family assessment and intervention by providing a framework to contextualize the numerous pieces of information that clinicians collect about client and family (Cox, in press; Fawcett, 1989). In working with families, professionals need to choose theories that best explain family situations and suggest effective goals and interventions (Fawcett, 1989; Grotevant, 1989).

Table 3.7.
Examples of Intervention Questions for the Seven Family Problem-Solving Steps

Problem-Solving Step	Type of Intervention Question	Intent of Question	Sample Questions
1. Identify the problem	Linear	Collect factual data	What has the doctor told you about your family member's condition?
		Define the family problem	Which of these problems is most troublesome for you?
2. Communicate with those involved	Linear	Determine who should be involved	Who else needs to know about your husband's problem?
	Strategic	Provide correct information	Child visiting is for ten minutes, so when can she be here?
3. Find alternate solutions	Strategic	Provide new information	Are you aware that your wife will be here two more weeks?
	Circular	Explore past and present coping patterns	When your husband was sick before, how did you manage?
	Reflexive	Explore possible solutions	Last time your neighbor looked after your children; can your sister do this now?
4. Choose a new solution	Strategic	Provide accurate information	When your father goes home, have you been told that you will need assistance?
	Reflexive	Facilitate new coping patterns	How will you manage to change your schedule, in order to care for your husband?
5. Implement a new solution	Linear	Inquire about new solution	Now that your sister is caring for the children, is this working out all right?
6. Observe outcomes of new solution	Circular	Explore how new solution has provided a new outcome	How has your change in child care affected your ability to visit your husband?
7. Evaluate effectiveness of new solution	Reflexive	Identify criteria to evaluate effectiveness of new solution	When you get discouraged, does it make you think you made the wrong choice?

Source: Davis and Cox (1995). Using interventive questions to empower family decision making. *Dimensions of Critical Care Nursing, 14*(1), 53. Copyright 2002 Lippincott Williams and Wilkins ©.

The Family Stress Theory-ABCX Model (Hill, 1965), Bowen's Family Systems Theory (1978), Olson's Circumplex Model of Family Functioning (Olson et al., 1985), and the Collaborative Language Systems Approach (H. Anderson, 1991a, 1991b; H. Anderson & Goolishian, 1988) are theoretical bases that can be useful for assessment and intervention. When these approaches are considered simultaneously with the Family Cycle of Health and Illness Model, the clinician will have a "full field of view" in understanding a family. The applications of each of these theories and models in a family interview is shown after each theory.

Family Stress Theory-ABCX Model

Hill (1949, 1958) identified a major set of variables and their relationships that led to family crisis. He named this The Family Stress Theory-ABCX Model. The Family Stress Theory is especially pertinent to health care situations due to the pervasive illness-related stresses that families experience (Artinian, 1994). The most amenable factor identified for nurse practitioner intervention is family stress (Murata, 1994). This two-part model explains what results in a crisis for one family and not another. The first part concerns the crisis determinants of A interacting with B interacting with C producing X where:

- A = family stressor—event/s and related hardships that may be so great as to change the family system
- B = family's crisis-meeting resources/coping mechanisms (i.e., religious faith, finances, social support, physical health, family flexibility, family coping mechanism)
- C = family's cognitive definition of event/s, how they deal with stressor/s, and family stress level: threatening = crisis, challenging = understandable and manageable
- X = family's level of disruption or incapacitation due to the stressor/s, resulting in crisis or noncrisis (Hill, 1965)

The second part concerns family adjustment after a crisis. Hill (1965) explained this adjustment as a period of disorganization, often seen in family relations and role performance, an upward angle of recovery, and reorganization and a new family functioning level. Crisis-prone families seem to have fewer resources and coping abilities. They fail to learn from experiences, seeing new stressors as threatening and crisis-provoking (Hill, 1965). McCubbin and McCubbin (1993) expanded on Hill's work and added "pile up of stressors." The number of demands on or within the family decides this along with "the trials and tribulations associated with the family's particular life-cycle stage with all of its demands and changes" (p. 28).

The following theoretical assumptions of the Family Stress Theory-ABCX Model provide justification for assessment and interventions with families:

1. Unexpected or unplanned events are usually perceived as stressful.
2. Lack of previous experience with stressor events leads to increased perceptions of stress.
3. Ambiguous stressor events are more stressful than nonambiguous events.

4. Events within families, i.e., serious illness, and defined as stressful, are more disruptive than stressors that occur outside the family, such as war, flood, or depression (Artinian, 1994).

Assessment areas cover the four prominent variables within the theory. Interventions include enhancement of family resources and support systems; modification of the family's perception of events rather than focus on the objective reality; and empowering families to recognize their resources and strengths. Interventions that bring forth past coping pattern use are easier than families learning new ways of responding.

Application

When talking with a family employing the ABCX Model, the clinician might ask the following questions: "How are each of you managing the grave news about your mother's illness?" (inquire how each person is managing as unexpected information is usually perceived as stressful); "How have you managed this type of serious illness in your family before?" (encourage helpful coping mechanism used in the past); "How are you dealing with this news about your mother?" (focus on the subjective perception rather than on the objective reality); and "What information do you need in order to understand and manage now?" (assist family in understanding and managing the situation).

Bowen Family Systems Theory

Family System Theory was developed by Bowen and is a well-recognized theory used to understand family functioning (Bowen, 1978; I. Goldenberg & Goldenberg, 1991; Kerr, 1981; Kerr & Bowen, 1988). Bowen's theory offers a natural systems theory in which the family is seen as an evolutionary process in nature (I. Goldenberg & Goldenberg, 1991). Bowen viewed the family as an emotional unit of interlocking relationships that is best understood within its multigenerational context.

According to Kerr (1981), Bowen's Family Systems Theory has eight interlocking concepts (see Table 3.8). Bowen's theory can provide clinicians with a framework for seeing all individual family members as being emotionally tied together in a thinking, feeling, and behavior relationship system across generations. The family genogram (see Figure 3.3) is a pictorial tool used by the clinician and family to understand family emotional processes in their multigenerational context (M. McGoldrick & Gerson, 1985).

Application

When talking with a family employing Bowen's family systems theory, the clinician might ask the following questions: "How did each of you in the family deal with Mary's death?" (differentiation of each family member); "Steve,

Table 3.8.
Bowen Family System Theory

Concept	Definition
1. Differentiation of self	The extent to which a person can distinguish between experienced intellectual and feeling processes
2. Triangles	At a certain intensity level, a third person is pulled into a relationship to dilute anxiety
3. Nuclear family emotional system	The fusion of the marital couple's emotional processes that will become unstable over time
4. Family projection process	Parents select the most infantile child as the object of their attention
5. Emotional cutoff	Flight from unresolved emotional ties with the family, not true emancipation
6. Multigenerational transmission process	Severe dysfunction as the result of the operation of the family emotional system over several generations
7. Sibling position	Interactive patterns between marital partners related to their position in the family of origin
8. Societal regression	Societal erosion of the forces intent on achieving individuation

when you and Gail are upset with each other, who do you talk to in the family?" (triangles); and "Gail, am I understanding you correctly that you left home when you were fourteen years old?" (emotional cutoff).

Olson Circumplex Model of Family Functioning

The Circumplex Model of Marital and Family Systems was developed to bridge the gaps that typically exist between research, theory, and practice (Olson, 1993; Olson et al., 1986). In this model, family cohesion, flexibility (originally called adaption), and communication are the three dimensions that developed from a conceptual clustering of more than fifty concepts that describe marital and family dynamics. *Family cohesion* is defined as "the emotional bonding that family members have toward one another" (p. 105) measured by concepts such as emotional bonding, boundaries, time, space, friends, and decision making. The four levels of cohesion range from disengaged (very low) to enmeshed (very high; see Figure 3.4). In a circumplex model, where most functional families are in the middle rather than at either

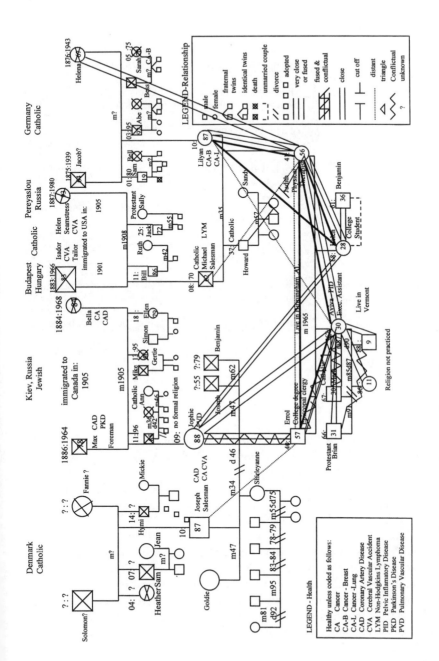

Figure 3.3. Transcultural Genogram (constructed in 1997)

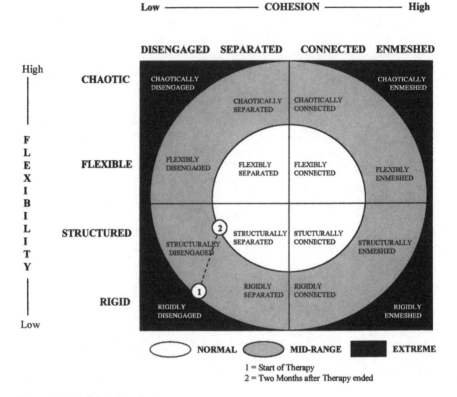

Figure 3.4. Belcher Family

extreme, the balanced area in the middle, separated and connected, indicates more functional families. Many troubled families that enter family therapy often fall into one of the extreme types.

Family flexibility is the amount of change in its leadership, role relationships, and relationship rules measured by concepts such as leadership, negotiation styles, role relationships, and relationship rules. The four levels of flexibility range from rigid (very low) to chaotic (very high; see Figure 3.4). Again, families within the central levels of the model "are more conducive to marital and family functioning" and are "more functional over time" (p. 107). Families that enter family therapy are often one of the extreme types. Family communication is considered a facilitating dimension, therefore it is not graphically displayed in the model. Research findings regarding communication and problem solving suggest that balanced family systems tend to have very good communication, whereas extreme family systems tend to have poor communication.

The model can be seen as a descriptive family map of sixteen family types—four levels of cohesion with four levels of flexibility (see Figure 3.4). The family map "is important because people often use their own family of origin as a reference for the type of marriage and family they either want or do not want" (Olson, 1993, p. 108). The model can be used to understand how the family develops across the family life cycle, changes within marital systems, and changes related to physical illness. The Family Adaptation and Cohesion Evaluation Scale–III (FACES–III; Olson et al., 1985) is a reliable and valid instrument based theoretically on the Circumplex Model to measure flexibility and cohesion. When working with clients in a clinical setting, FACES–III should be used for assessment and continued care rather than FACES–II, which is more appropriate when conducting research (L. Knutson-Life Innovations, Inc., personal communication, December 17, 2001). Scores obtained from FACES–III are plotted on the model. For reliability and validity data on FACES–III, see Olson, 1993; Olson et al., 1986. Clinically, FACES–III can be used to determine a family's current level of functioning and to guide treatment planning and interventions to promote more functional family patterns. The instrument can be used at various points in treatment to measure family dynamics (see Figure 3.4).

Application

When working with a family employing the Circumplex Model, the clinician might ask the following questions related to cohesion: "How would your family describe how close they feel to one another?" (emotional bonding); "How easy is it for your children's friends to come over 'any old time'?" (boundaries); and "How do you make decisions in your family?" (decision making); and these questions related to flexibility: "Who would you say is the leader of your family?" (leadership); "How does your family negotiate differences?" (negotiation styles); and "What are the rules about how your children speak to you?" (relationship rules).

Collaborative Language Systems Approach

The Collaborative Language Systems Approach takes social construction theory and applies it to therapeutic work with clients. This approach views human beings as language-generating, meaning-generating systems engaged in social conversations that are constantly changing, creative, and dynamic (H. Anderson, 1991a, 1991b; see Table 3.9). Human systems are seen as existing in the domain of language and its meaning. Language refers to meaning that is generated between people through the medium of words and other communicative actions that result in a shared reality (H. Anderson, 1997; H. Anderson & Goolishian, 1988). However, no communication or word is complete, clear, and univocal. All words carry unspoken meanings and possible new interpretations that require expression and articulation. In this area of "the unexpressed" lies the opportunity for evolutionary change in meaning. Inherent in this view is an appreciation for the expertise that each client has on his or her life, that

Table 3.9.
Collaborative Language Systems Approach

Foundational Premises for Possibility Conversations

A. Human systems are language-generating and, simultaneously, meaning-generating systems. Communication and discourse define social organizations (i.e., a sociocultural system is the product of social communication rather than communication being a product of organization). Hence, any human system is a linguistic or communicative system. The therapeutic system is a linguistic system.

B. Meaning and understanding are socially and intersubjectively constructed. By intersubjective, we refer to an evolving state of affairs in which two or more people agree (understand) that they are experiencing the same event in the same way. Meaning and understanding involve this intersubjective experience. However, it is understood that agreement is fragile and continually open to renegotiation and dispute. We do not arrive at or have meaning and understanding until we take communicative action, that is, engage in some meaning generating discourse or dialogue within a system for which the communication has relevance. A therapeutic system is a system for which the communication has a relevance specific to itself.

C. Any therapeutic system is one that has coalesced around some "problem" - the relevance - and will be engaged in evolving language and meaning specific to itself, specific to its organization and specific to its dis-solution around "the problem." In this sense, the therapeutic system is a system that is distinguished by "the problem" rather than a social structure that distinguishes "the problem." The therapeutic system is a problem-organizing, problem-dis-solving system.

D. Therapeutic intervention is a linguistic event that takes place in what we call a therapeutic conversation. The therapeutic conversation is a mutual search and exploration through dialogue, a two-way exchange, a crisscrossing of ideas in which new meanings are continually evolving toward the "dis-solving" of problems and, thus, the dissolving of the therapy system and, hence, the problem-organizing, problem-dis-solving system. Change is the evolution of new meaning through dialogue.

Table 3.9.
Continued

E.   The role of the clinician is that of a master conversational artist--an architect of dialogue

whose expertise is in <u>creating a space for</u> and <u>facilitating</u> a dialogical conversation. The

therapist is a participant-observer and a conversational-partner of the therapeutic

conversation.

Source: Adapted from H. Anderson and Goolishian (1988); H. Anderson (1997).

each client has the resources for his or her problem's solution, and that most clients strive for healthy relationships and successful lives. When assuming this view, clinicians act and talk in ways that create a space for and invite relationships and conversations where clients and clinicians connect, collaborate, and construct with each other.

Therapeutic interactions with clients and their families is a process of expressing and expanding what has been "the unsaid." The clinician's role is that of a conversational partner, referring to conversation characterized as a two-way conversation, back-and-forth, give-and-take, in-there-together process in which people talk with each other rather than to each other. Inviting this kind of partnership requires a belief that the client's story takes center stage. Listening interactively refers to the continual process of checking out that the clinician is understanding the client from the client's perspective. This clinician role and activity invite the client and family into a mutual or shared inquiry in which the clinician and client coexplore the familiar and codevelop the new. The conversational partnership creates a sense of belonging for the client and family, inviting participation and shared responsibility for its outcome. Through this dialogue come new ideas, themes, and narratives that create new solutions that are individually tailored to the client's need. In this manner of interacting in brief, episodic encounters, clinicians can empower families to create new solutions to their present problems (Cox & Davis, 1993).

Application

As the clinician and family continue to dialogue, the Collaborative Language Systems Approach suggests the following questions: "Steve and Gail, I noticed that one of the problems you all mentioned several days ago was your sexual relationship, yet you have not talked about it. How could we talk about your sexual relationship?" (area of "the unexpressed"); "Steve, I have an idea that you have some thoughts about the relationship between Gail and your mother, Mary, that you have not shared with us. What would need to happen for you to talk about those ideas here?" (creates a space for constructive dialogue); and

"Gail, what have you been able to do that has been helpful to you in dealing with Mary's death that you have not talked with Steve about?" (meaning and understanding are socially and intersubjectively constructed).

Reflecting Team Approach When Working with Families

Andersen (1987) is credited with beginning work with families using a "reflecting team" (p. 415). This occurred when he was supervising a young family interviewer who repeatedly got seduced by the family into having the same pessimism about the family as the family had about itself. With permission of the family, the family viewed a conversation between the supervisors behind the mirror after which the interview proceeded in a more optimistic view.

Much of Andersen's work is built on an understanding of Bateson's (1972, 1979) and Maturana's (1978; Maturana & Varela, 1980) view of epistemology—that is, the reality we know is created within us and therefore each person has their own reality. Thus, there is a both–and or neither–nor not an either/ or. Maturana believes that living entities are structurally determined, that is, they can operate only out of and in accord with the way they are built. Therefore, systems have a way of functioning with many parts in their repertory that help them adapt to the environment. One part, whether a group or person, must remember that the other part can only participate through one of the modes of relating that is already available in its repertory. "If the relationship between the parts is 'safe' enough, nonintrusive enough, interesting enough, the mutual exchanges that carry new ideas may trigger new modes of relating" (Andersen, 1987, p. 416).

The task of the reflecting team is to create new ideas among the three persons on the team. The ideas of the team are to be presented in a manner that will be best received by the family—safe enough to be considered part of the family system. The team ideally will match the style of the family, "their rhythm, speed, and modes of communication" (p. 421), and take into account the cultural/ ethical aspects of the family. For example, in Andersen's country of Norway, Norwegians speak slowly, therefore, the reflecting team works slowly.

The reflections should have the quality of tentative suggestions, not pronouncements, interpretations, or supervisory remarks. For example, the ideas may start with, "I am not sure . . . ," "It could be that . . . ," "Maybe . . . ," "Maybe this does not fit but. . . ." The hope is that the suggested ideas will trigger a small change in the family's view of the problem or in its understanding of the problem. However, the ideas presented by the team may not be of any interest to the family or the family may completely disagree with the team members' ideas. All is not lost if this occurs. This, in and of itself, will create new dialogue for the family and the interviewer. The team can then create alternative explanations for the problem and discuss what should remain the same and what must be changed. Eventually there can be dialogue about what the understandings are within the family that hold the family together in a stuck place and what can be changed enough to make a difference. In all discussions with the family, the team must remain "positive, discreet, respectful, sensitive, imaginative, and creatively free" (p. 424). If the family is indiscreet in betraying more than they wished to be known, the reflecting team must reply with a protective carefulness when responding to the family.

COUNSELING POINTS

- Family health counseling incorporates and intersects all levels of the family, community, and society.

- Interaction, circularity, and reciprocity guide clinicians view of families' reflexive relationships.

- Clinicians must assess if working with the whole family is appropriate presently.

- Families are always at different points on the health–illness continuum.

- Clinicians must adopt a theoretical stance that both supports the clinician's view and provides family care at all levels of the family, community, and society.

- Collaboration with families assists them is utilizing their own self-agency.

- Reflecting teams assist both clinicians and families in meeting the family's goals.

4

Sociocultural Influences on the Family and Family Health

Ruth P. Cox, Sylvia London, Irma Punsky, Conchita Quiroz, Rocio Martinez Zaid, and Alberto Díaz

THE COMPLEX CULTURAL CONTEXT AND ITS CHANGING SALIENCE

The broad definition of culture emphasizes inclusion rather than exclusion, recognizes that each of us belongs to many different cultures at the same time, and further recognizes that these many potential cultural identities take turns in being salient according to changing circumstances. Culture becomes the totality of what each person has learned from every other person. The visual image is of being surrounded by more than 1,000 "culture teachers" that have been gathered from friends, enemies, heros, heroines, and fantasies one's whole life. All behaviors are learned in this cultural context and are displayed in a cultural context. Consequently, accurate assessment, meaningful understanding, and appropriate therapeutic intervention must attend to that cultural context. Individual differences of skin color, intelligence, height, and genetic potentials take on cultural meaning through interacting with other people and learning the rules of one's different cultures. These ideas are certainly supported by Constantine, Juby, and Liang (2001). In their recent research, these authors suggested that "without raising awareness about the impact of their [therapists'] own worldviews in counseling situations," therapists "may not be fully cognizant of the ways in which they may impose Eurocentric thoughts, expectations, and behaviors in the context of therapeutic relationships" (p. 359).

In *transcultural counseling*, it is important to examine each behavior in its cultural context. Behavior is not meaningful data until and unless it is understood in the context of the person's culturally learned expectations. This allows clinicians to identify common ground between two culturally different people whose positive expectations and ultimate goals—for trust, respect, or success— are the same even though behaviors may vary. Even the same individuals may change their cultural referent group from emphasizing gender to age to SES or ethnicity or something else in the same interview. The transcultural family clinician must be skilled in understanding the changing salience of all potential cultural identities. This makes it possible to reframe conflict between parent and child, husband and wife, or brother and sister that might not otherwise be considered "cultural" so that each person's behavior is understood in the context of his or her expectations and values. If two people share the same positive expectation, they do not have to display the same behaviors to find common ground.

For example, smiling is an ambiguous behavior. It may imply trust and friendliness or it may not. The smile may be interpreted accurately or it may not be. Outside its cultural context, the smile has no fixed meaning. Two persons may both expect trust and friendliness even though one is smiling and the other is not. If these similar positive expectations are undiscovered or disregarded, then behavioral differences may result in conflict. This makes it imperative that the meaning of behavior is understood through the lens of the cultures involved. If, however, two culturally different persons understand how they perhaps really have the same positive expectations even though their behaviors may be different, a positive outcome is possible (Pedersen, 1997).

BICULTURAL AND MULTICULTURAL FAMILIES

All families are bicultural or multicultural but not all families are aware of the consequence of defining culture broadly. Attempts to change behaviors in the family will necessarily look at the different and changing roles that each family member assumes in the family interaction. This will be inclusive of the positive and negative contribution of those roles to the family. The family system becomes more than the sum of its parts or members in ways typical to interacting systems. Butz (1997) described the applications of chaos theory and complexity theory to family therapy. Chaos and complexity theory look at the nonlinear and self-regulating variables that lead to unpredictability in complex relationships. Each system shares responsibility for mutual causality as an interdependent member. Open systems such as families have a continuously changing flow of power characterized by interaction and connections among family members as relationships and patterns are repeated or changed. The clinician attempts to redirect or influence those changes in functionally healthy directions by recognizing each behavior and each change in the larger sociocultural context.

Not all families are willing or able to deal with their complex, dynamic cultural context. When the salient difference is ethnicity or nationality, the bicultural factor becomes more obvious. Yet the same dynamics occur in families that are not so obviously bicultural or multicultural. Each family is a sociocultural system that has its own unique rules and roles. Each family has an organized power structure at the overt and covert levels and special "insider ways" of negotiating and problem solving. Each family has a shared history that gives deep meaning to underlying assumptions and loyalties. By conceptualizing these differences as cultural, it is possible for two family members to disagree in their behaviors without either one being wrong, as long as they can discover a common ground of shared positive expectations in their family cultural context.

INCREASING EMPHASIS ON NON-WESTERN APPROACHES

Although "Western" cultures emphasize individualism, "non-Western" cultures emphasize collectivism as a core value. The family functions quite differently in an individualist society compared to a collectivist society. Individualists have more personal choice in their careers, memberships, religious affiliations, political affiliations, and social roles. Individualists can and do change roles or affiliations more frequently. They are free to choose which family members to stay in contact with and how close that contact will be. In collectivist societies, a person's group memberships are more fixed. One's family of origin specifies the roles one is required to take in life (Bond, 1994). A Westernized description of the family presumes a separate, independent, and autonomous group guided by traits, abilities, values, and motives that distinguish each family from others. Western cultures are described by Berry, Poortinga, Segall, and Dansen (1992) as more "idiocentric," emphasizing competition, self-confidence, and freedom, whereas collectivistic cultures are more allocentric, emphasizing communal responsibility, social usefulness, and acceptance of authority.

Both Western and non-Westernized approaches to the family emphasize development. Non-Western systems focus on development with a transpersonal focus of well-being, whereas Western systems focus on psychopathology and measured physical and mental changes. Western models tend to pathologize mystical experiences, whereas non-Western models tend to pathologize self-serving behaviors of family members. Increased attention to non-Western approaches have resulted from international contact and some dissatisfaction with the disruptive influences of individualism. Family complexity has inhibited research on cultural aspects of family functioning. "Given the lack of theory in academic psychology to throw light on family functioning and family change, the prototypical Western (middle-class, nuclear) family has been adopted implicitly as the family" (Kagitcibasi, 1996, p.73). The shift of global socioeconomic development toward traditionally collectivistic societies is likely to increase the attention given to collectivisitic views. Therefore, clinicians must attend to these different views when assessing the functional status of the family.

TRANSCULTURAL ASSESSMENT MODEL

In response to the need for a practical assessment tool for evaluating cultural variables and their effects on health and illness behaviors, Giger and Davidhizar (1995) created the Transcultural Assessment Model. They emphasized that as "every individual is culturally unique," health care providers "must use caution to avoid projecting on the client their own 'cultural uniqueness' and 'world views,' if culturally appropriate care is to be provided" (p. 8). Knowledge of culturally relevant information can assist in planning and implementing a treatment regimen that is unique for families while incorporating their cultural context.

The Transcultural Assessment Model provides a systemic approach to evaluating six essential cultural phenomena when providing culturally appropriate care. "Although the six cultural phenomena are evident in all cultural groups, they vary in application across cultures" (Giger & Davidhizar, 1995, p. 9). Figure 4.1 lists the six phenomena. An individualized assessment is necessary when working with families with diverse cultural heritages as cultural variations among populations dictate unique treatment implications (Degazon, 1996). For example, consider the cultural variable of communication. A clinician, while being careful not to stereotype, would not be surprised by individuals with a Russian heritage using touch freely with family members and close friends (Giger & Davidhizar, 1995, see p. 373). This type of communication in the family would be usual for individuals with this cultural heritage. If observed, the clinician could inquire about how this is helpful to the family. If not there, the clinician could inquire what communication has taken its place and how this has occurred from generation through generation. Degazon (1996), Grossman (1996), and Giger and Davidhizar (1995) provided other examples of cultural variations for each of the six phenomena.

The Transcultural Family approach (Figure 4.2) views families through the lens of culture while considering both internal and external forces that can affect family functioning. These forces are understood using theories or paradigms, such as Bowen's, Olson's or Anderson's, and concepts, such as structure,

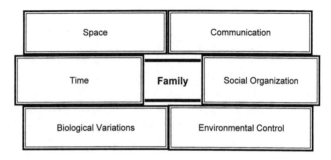

Figure 4.1. Transcultural Organizers

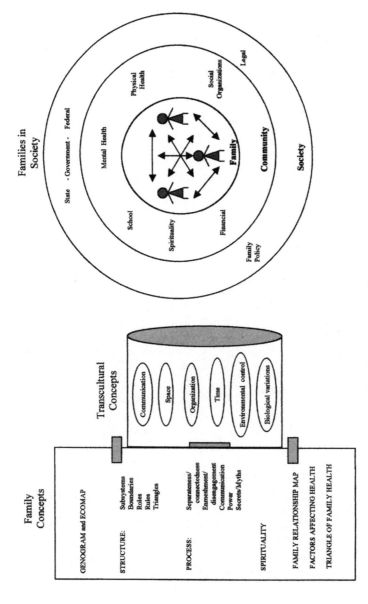

Figure 4.2. Concepts Used with Families from Diverse Cultures

process, spirituality, and the Triangle of Family Health. The process includes assessment, using the Family Health and Functioning Assessment, a treatment plan, interventions, including specific therapist skills, and evaluation. During treatment, these phases weave back and forth, in and out, recursively. As new information is discovered, new plans are made, and intervention and evaluation guide future phases.

Case Study: Hispanic/Mexican Heritage

Using Giger and Davidhizar's Transcultural Assessment Model, the following is an actual case seen at a public children's hospital in Mexico. The family was seen through the Family Therapy Department at a hospital by a team formed of master's level students in their fifth-semester clinical practicum and their supervisors. Given the specific characteristics of the training program at the university, the hospital, and the family, the team was dealing with at least three different systems, merging in a treatment session. In addition to the three identified systems, each with its own organizing beliefs, all team members had their own individual set of beliefs and ideas within the treatment team.

The Team

The team was new in this training/teaching hospital and the team's particular way of working was not known or trusted by the hospital staff. Yet the team continued to receive referrals. At first, the team addressed the "hospital culture" that had to do with their presence in the facility and their personal and professional relationships with the hospital staff. In order to adapt their work to the hospital, a reporting style was developed according to the institution and hospital rules. These adaptations emphasized the transcultural phenomena of communication style, time, space, and social organization.

The team's postmodern/social constructionist approach, as used in H. Anderson's (1997) Collaborative Language Systems Approach, was not familiar to the hospital staff. They were, however, familiar with systemic family therapy and reflecting teams. Therefore, the team used these familiar lenses to describe their work to provide a common ground of shared positive expectations and experiences within the staff's cultural context. Their work was made public and open to any member of the staff interested in visiting their work and participating with the team.

As the team worked with families, they invited families to visit the "team's culture" of therapy that included different transcultural phenomena of communication styles, space usage, time management, and different organization. The team described, explained, and presented their working guidelines—the team consisted of two therapists (male and female) who worked with the family in the room while the reflecting team assisted from behind the one-way mirror. Once the family became familiarized with the team's proposal, the team was then ready to enter the "family's culture."

Family Identifying Information

Tania is a sixteen-year-old Hispanic/Mexican female who had been admitted to the hospital's adolescent girls unit due to a suicide attempt. She was referred to the Family Therapy Unit by the hospital following her stay on the adolescent unit. Tania lived with her mother; her seventeen-year-old brother; and Miguel, an uncle who was disabled (mentally retarded) and an alcoholic. There were no other health problems within the family. The family was Catholic in their religious beliefs but their priest was not involved with family during their treatment. Tania, her mother, and Miguel attended the first meeting. Tania's parents had been divorced for some years, yet the family still kept some contact with their father. Tania had left her school when she was admitted to the hospital. Tania was described by her brother as "stubborn, spoiled, aggressive, angry and irresponsible." Tania's mother believed that Tania's behavior was the result of the sexual abuse she had suffered by her grandfather.

Presenting Problem

After a long fight with her mother, Tania took pills with the intention of killing herself. She was taken to the hospital for treatment and then referred to the inpatient unit for psychiatric and psychological assessment and treatment. Tania was sexually abused by her paternal grandfather from ages six to twelve. At the time, Tania's grandparents lived with Tania's family. When Tania was twelve years old, she disclosed the abuse to her mother. Subsequently, the grandfather disappeared and within three months, the grandmother died of diabetes. At the time the team began treatment, Tania was using cocaine. She and her mother were already receiving group therapy at an addiction center and both were in individual treatment.

Assessment Phase

The teamwork approach included two therapists in the room and a reflecting team behind the mirror. The assessment and the first cultural interaction became one. In the initial contact, the team introduced themselves and gathered some family information to help generate more ideas for their particular situation. The questions were asked in a very friendly and open manner, but at the same time reflected the preference in Mexican culture for a closer and more familiar way of relating. Very early on in treatment, Tania's mother commented about the therapist's age, being young, and saw that as an asset, along with the team's curiosity and genuine concern for the family story and dilemmas. As the male in the family, Miguel came for the first session, as this had been a family tradition. Culturally, this action could be seen as making sure the women of the family were in a safe place. Being convinced of their safety, he did not feel the need to come back, despite the team's suggestions and requests.

Treatment Plan

The team decided to see the family every other week and discussed this with the family. This arrangement was suitable to the family in terms of time, space, and budget. In this initial joining, the therapists had to be careful to address Tania as she had been seen as oppositional. The therapists spent time alone with Tania and together they decided the meetings could continue with Tania and her mother in the same room.

The therapists and team based their assumptions on the notion of change and possibilities (O'Hanlon & Weiner-Davis, 1989). The team believed that this family wanted to change and that they had the resources to do so (focusing on the future). Tania's mother and brother believed, and mentioned, that all the problems came from Tania's childhood abuse. The team kept coming back to this issue as often as needed (focusing on the past). On the other hand, the therapists decided not to dwell on the abuse, from the idea that one does not have to understand the cause or origin of a problem in order to solve it. On the contrary, they focused on resources and positive experiences.

Here, the team faced the difference between the family, who culturally tended to be past–present-oriented, and the therapist preference toward the future. Given the cultural preferences, the team kept honoring the family's needs, but at the same time looked at the possibilities toward the future. The team was able to combine storytelling that had to do with the family's past, while simultaneously staying focused on the changes toward the future.

Intervention

The family was seen for seven sessions that lasted approximately one hour. Each session was conducted in this order: presession; family session; intersession, usually behind the mirror with the reflecting team; and closing family session, where sometimes team members were invited to participate.

At the third session, Tania announced to the therapist that she had made the decision to stop using cocaine and to start working. These changes, which seemed to be so sudden, were not surprising. The team expected change, embraced it, and did not question it.

An intervention, taken from narrative therapies (White & Epston, 1980), consisted of a letter written by the therapists and given to Tania and her family at the last session (a translation to English from the Spanish original):

Let's finish with you Tania. First we would like to tell you that we are very impressed by all the changes you have made in such a short time, this is quite unusual, young lady. At sixteen, to be able to leave the drugs behind, to acknowledge and recognize the risks along the way and to know what works for you and what is useless, will help you build your own life project. It looks like nobody knows your resources better that you do. You have found a job that suits your professional interest and you have found a way to create a team with your family. You know that your way of solving your life dilemmas has changed, if in the past you used to direct your anger towards yourself or others, now you have realized that everything takes time and that words are at your service to face any situation as difficult as it might look.

Reflecting Team

As mentioned earlier, a reflecting team was used, which was an adapted version of the ideas introduced by Andersen (1987) and his colleagues in Norway. Given the space constraints, the team used a one-way mirror and had some discussions behind the mirror, some in front of the family, and at other times, reflecting team members were invited to share their ideas directly with the family. At the beginning, the situation was new for the family, but they liked it. They said that listening to the team's conversations helped them think about the problem in and out of the sessions in ways that they hadn't thought before. They became so familiar with the reflecting team members that they knew their names, wanted to know who was there, and on some occasions asked for a specific team member to give her opinion on a particular topic. The family also expressed their desire to be in touch with the treatment team in the future if the occasion called for further meetings.

Adaptions of the reflecting team were made that reflected directly the culture it was entering. The family became close, attached, and related in a very friendly and familiar way to the team members. The reflecting team members, in general, spoke directly to the family members or to the therapist. The team was careful to listen to the clients and to honor their request when they wanted a specific team member to participate in the reflections. The family took care of the therapist and their learning situation and were concerned about how useful they were being because they were all learning together in front of this team. Following are the family's reflections on the team's participation in the process:

The surprise was to have another view . . . the conversations you had there . . . and then when you entered the room and talked among themselves (team) and you (therapists) here . . . is a different system, but it works like a mirror. (Mother and Tania)

We felt we had more support, in sharing with other people, in not being afraid to be exposed. (Mother)

There were more people listening to me . . . I like it. (Tania)

Evaluation

The general attitude and philosophy of work was based on the collaborative language approach and the work of H. Anderson (1997), which led to a "not knowing position," developing a sense of agency, curiosity, and following of the client's lead. The family's testimonies regarding this kind of work might be the best way to assess the possibility of conveying this attitude and posture in a therapeutic setting. The family's evaluation of their experience in therapy follow (this is translated verbatim from Spanish):

About the therapists . . .

It is important to know that we are in the presence of people whose work is not to tell us what to do or how to do it, but to provide other views and ways to understand our attitudes, actions and solve our problems in the best possible way . . . (Mother)

About the sense of personal agency . . .

I feel very happy, because we all, in our own personal way and style, worked to save our home, I mean all of us even the father and Miguel. (Mother)

The decisions were taken by me. (Tania)

We already learned to converse and to give us time to think and reflect. We already built this path and it will be very difficult to get out of it. (Mother)

About the process . . .

. . . something that arrived here shapeless got some shape and form through the trust and the atmosphere, something that we slowly built. It was like giving shape to these situations that make us lose sight of the vision, the dimension, the limits . . . is something. . . . I was so lost. (Mother)

It is great. (Tania)

What was different . . .

The way you ask questions . . . the first psychologist I went to see . . . I did not like to go . . . she had an ugly way of asking . . . not here . . . psychology is great. (Tania)

Advice for the therapists . . .

It was great . . . we slowly became sure of ourselves, keep the freshness you have, this possibility to develop trust, to be with us to compliment us, to be part of the team, to be close to our problems and dilemmas . . . from the first day I did not feel that you were out there like therapists, you were right here like people. (Mother and Tania)

Conclusions

This particular case gave the team the luxury of entering the family's experience in therapy through their own words and personal experience. The team witnessed how the social constructionist approach in therapy allows them to address the cultural needs in a way that honored and respected the individual variables. These variables were highlighted by Giger and Davidhizar's Transcultural Assessment Model that include communication, time, space, social organization, environmental control, and biological variables. The therapists and the clients joined in creating a treatment system where they were able to explore the familiar and develop the newness in a respectful, caring, and familiar environment.

RACE, ETHNICITY, AND FAMILY DEVELOPMENT

Race is primarily a social classification that relies on physical markers, such as skin color, facial feature, and hair texture to identify group membership. Families may be of the same race, but may differ in ethnic affiliations. Although families who are of one race may be heterogeneous in their origin, they are often viewed as ethnically and racially homogenous. On the other hand, ethnicity is based on individuals and families sharing the similar values, beliefs, customs, religion, behavior and traditions—a common ancestry. Ethnicity is influenced by education, location, income, social class, and associations with others outside the families' group—thus there are different levels of ethnicity within the same ethnic group. A frequent consequence of these views and levels of ethnicity is that cultural and ethnic difference is often obscured or suppressed in favor of racial characteristics (Snowden & Holschuh, 1992). Thus, the cultural and ethnic diversity of the family is blurred and lost. Conversely, in biracial and multiracial families where family development over multiple generations has led to changes in physical appearance, race is seen as less important than ethnic identity.

Now, however, clinicians are more often appreciating that variations in family structure and family development of different races (i.e., African Americans, Asians, Hispanics, Whites, and others) are potentially strengths in helping families to function under various economic and social conditions (Wright & Leahey, 2000). Racial differences, in and of themselves, are not a problem per se. Rather the problems related to race are those of prejudice, stereotyping, discrimination, ethnocentrism, cultural imposition, and other types of intercultural aggression based on difference. Many health-related associations have position statements related to this. For example, The American Nurses Association's (2001) has a Position Statement on Cultural Diversity in Nursing Practice as follows, "Ethnocentric approaches to nursing practice are ineffective in meeting health and nursing needs of diverse cultural groups of clients." It is important for clinicians to understand family health beliefs and behaviors, influenced by racial identity, privilege, or oppression, as it effects family development and health care practices (Wright & Leahey, 2000).

ETHNIC AND CULTURAL DIVERSITY AND SOCIAL CLASS DISPARITIES IN THE UNITED STATES

Ethnic and Cultural Diversity

Since the 1960s, there has been a steady growth in the racial and ethnic diversity (also called cultural diversity) of the United States. The White majority is aging and decreasing, while there is an increase in the population of African American, Hispanic American, Asian and Pacific Islander American, and Native American populations (U.S. Census, 1992e). During the 1980–1990 decade there was more than a 100% increase in several racial/ethnic groups such as Chinese 104.1%, Asian Indian 125.3%, Korean 125.3%, and Vietnamese 134.8% (U.S. Census, 1983, 1992e). Other groups had increases of more than 50% such as Samoan 50.1%, Guamanian 53.4%, Mexican, 54.4%, and Other Hispanic 66.7%.

This increase in the diversity of the U.S. population led to an ever more complex cultural diversity when the demographics of groups were examined. For instance, the Asian American populations bring to the United States "at least 23 subgroups such as Asian Indian, Cambodian, Chinese, Filipino, Hmong, Japanese, Korean, Lotian, Thai, Vietnamese, and 'other Asian,' with 32 linguistic groups" (Inouye, 1999, p. 338). In addition to linguistic differences, this group shares many cultural characteristics that have been influenced by different religions, such as Buddhism, Confucianism, and Taoism.

The U.S. population growth is overwhelmingly due to a growth within racial and ethnic minority populations. Between 1980 and 1990, the Anglo-American percent of the population fell from 83.2% to 80.3%, whereas the percent for all other groups within the United States grew from 16.8% to 19.7% (U.S. Census, 1983, Tables 38 & 39; 1992e-Table 3). Some states seem to be centers for immigration into the United States, such as California, Illinois, and New York.

Social Class Disparities

During the 1980s and early 1990s, the rich continued to increase their wealth and the poor continued to become poorer (Peterson, 1993; Wolff, 1995). This disparity has been exacerbated by escalating national debt, a sluggish economy, increasing unemployment rates, and declining wages. The disparity in economic income made it difficult for lower class and working-class families to have access to employment and education. Thus, middle-class families decreased and families at both ends of the income continuum increased (i.e., increased numbers of rich and poor families). Economic recovery in the latter 1990s led to some growth in domestic programs, although the effects of the decline are still evident.

Economic inequality and reduction in social policy and health programs for the poor affected the health and health care of families. "Unequal distribution of preventive and basic health care resources results in morbidity and mortality rates that vary significantly between white people and nonwhite people and among socioeconomic class" (Hanson, 2001, p. 106). The health status of poor Americans is poorer than other social classes. For example, babies of poor families, regardless of racial or ethnic heritage, die two times as often as those in families who are not poor (P. Lee & Estes, 1997).

INFLUENCE OF CULTURAL AND SOCIAL CLASS ON FAMILY HEALTH WITHIN THE FAMILY AND IN HEALTH CARE SETTINGS

Family Influence on Family Health

Culture, passed down through multiple generations, influences the health status of the family over time. Culture provides a model of health and illness, which includes beliefs about what a symptom is, what it means, when and where you go for treatment, what symbolizes relief or cure, and what are the health practices that go along with family developmental events, such as child birth. These health beliefs are translated into health care practices that then affect the family health status. Examples of culturally derived values that can influence family health are: setting priorities for decision making, ability to deal with illness, value of relationships—individual versus family, time orientation—present versus future, and relationship to the community—congruence between family and community. "What constitutes appropriate care for specific health conditions is bound by cultural and social class expectations" (Hanson & Boyd, 1996, p. 87).

Western cultures typically root the explanation of health and illness in natural phenomena and scientific findings, whereas in non-Western societies families may understand illness as resulting from social or supernatural causes or from unbalances (hot and cold) in the body. Effective therapy is directly related to the cause—if the cause of the illness is spiritual, then prayers and other spiritual interventions are used. The cultural health heritage can be influenced by the amount of acculturation that has occurred within the family. The dominant culture may have influence on the family's health behaviors, such that different generations may have different views of what the family health behaviors should be. This continuum ranges from adhering to traditional cultural health values to adopting the health care practices of the dominant culture.

Social class status is strongly correlated with the ability of a family to maintain its health. "The more affluent an individual or family, the better life conditions, the greater their access to preventive and curative health care services, and the better their health status" (Hanson & Boyd, 1996, p. 92). Also, families from the upper and middle classes, whatever their ethnic heritage, tend to have better self-care health behaviors. In the United States, more than 11% of families live in poverty—this equates to 35.6 million people living below the poverty level (U.S. Bureau of the Census, 1998). Due to numerous stressors, the poor and underclass find it difficult to be future-oriented and concerned about healthy lifestyle choices. This also applies to children. Starfield (1992) found that poor children are more likely to become ill and have serious illnesses than children from higher income families. Poor children have more exposure to environmental hazards, poor nutrition, inadequate preventive care, and poor access to medical care—all social class inequalities. Research findings since the 1930s consistently show that lower class, economically distressed families are more likely to have poorer family health, less family stability, poorer marital adjustment, fewer family coping skills, and more troubled family relationships (Voydanoff & Donnelly, 1988).

Health Professionals' Influence on Family Health

Cultural differences may often be at the root of poor communication, avoidance of working well with others, interpersonal tensions, and inadequate assessment of health problems and their treatment. When differences exist between the clinician and the family, health care practices may not be based on the patient's needs (Sue & Sue, 1990). Clinicians always must be open to, and ever curious about, the variety of cultural differences among families, while not stereotyping families based on their cultural heritage. Health-seeking behaviors are determined by the family's customs, folk remedies, values, and beliefs. What families view as health, illness, crisis, and resources vary according to their cultural, racial, and ethnic heritage. This heritage can be influenced over time and generations by the amount of acculturation (the increasing similarity of two cultures) that has occurred, so that several generations who may even live within the same household may have very different views. Whether families live in rural or urban communities can also affect the erosion of cultural patterns over time.

When dealing with problems or illness in the family, clinicians have often dismissed social class issues to be of "little consequence to the 'serious talk' about illness" (Wright & Leahey, 2000, p. 84). This allows clinicians to sidestep many class issues related to inequality and injustice. Family treatment must take into account the cultural, ethnic, social, and economic context in which the family lives. Therefore, successful health care of families of diverse cultural, ethnic, and social backgrounds is dependent on the clinician's cultural competence in providing care for families from diverse cultures.

INTERACTION OF CULTURE AND SOCIAL CLASS: EFFECTS ON FAMILY HEALTH

While the influences of culture and social class individually on family health are considerable, the influence of the two together are profound (Hanson, 2001). Certain groups within the United States live in poverty largely due to ethnic and/or racial inequalities and social stratification. Families of color and ethnic families are much more likely to be poor than White families of European decent. Kliman (1998) noted that in a racist and classist society, class and race are not inseparable. For example, because poverty is disproportionately concentrated among racial minorities, many professionals have considered the African American statistical subgroup to represent the lower income class and the White statistical subgroup to represent the middle to upper income class group (Wright & Leahey, 2000). Moreover, "Much of the literature confounds the effects of race and class, not to mention the 'myth of sameness' about families within each race or class" (p. 83).

Being poor and being from an ethnic family of color position both individuals and families to sustain greater health hazards than being either from an ethnic family of color that is not poor or from a poor White family (Hanson, 2001). Reasons for this include differing access to health services and health insurance, differing exposure to health hazards, and differing family lifestyle practices. P. Lee and Estes (1997) suggested that major indicators of health status clearly demonstrate that minority Americans have a substantially poorer status than that of White Americans. Anglo-American children are four times less likely to live in poverty than African American and Hispanic children (U.S. Bureau of the Census, 1997). Furthermore, these poor minority children have more indicators of poorer health status. As ethnically diverse families are more often disadvantaged socioeconomically as well, these factors have a significant impact on the family's ability to influence its health status (Cockerham, 1987). Of these two factors, being poor is a greater detriment to obtaining health care services (Spector, 1996). Lack of health insurance is another major barrier to obtaining health care according to a national survey of health care and health insurance coverage. For example, de la Torre (1993) suggested that almost 40% of working-age Latinos have no health insurance.

Family health care practices are also influenced by culture and social class. Ethnic families who are poor may use folk medicine and home remedies more often than they would prefer as they lack access to health care (de la Torre, 1993). Keefe (1981) showed that middle and upper class Mexican-Americans seldom used folk medicine, whereas it was used frequently among lower class families. Contrary to this, Miller (1990) found that Korean families used Eastern medical treatments (herb and acupuncture) regardless of income or education. Higher income families used herbal medicines more often than poor families. This may have been due to the expense of the herbal medications and poor families could not afford them.

COUNSELING POINTS

- Individual differences take on cultural meaning through interaction with others.
- Families function differently in a individualist society than in a collectivist society.
- Clinicians can use a transcultural model to work with families from various cultures.
- Increased cultural diversity = need for more culturally competent clinicians.
- Social class is strongly correlated with family health maintenance.
- Poor, ethnic families may use home remedies/folk medicine as first line of defense.

5

Family Health Issues

Ruth P. Cox and Ken Farr

FAMILY HEALTH DEFINED

In reviewing the literature concerning family health, it is clear that the concept is consistently less well defined than the concept of health. It is usually defined according to the discipline and the theoretical framework that is used to define it. For example, family scientists define a healthy family as resilient (McCubbin & McCubbin, 1993) as well as possessing a balance of cohesion and flexibility that is facilitated by communication (Olson, 1993). Family therapy defines family health according to the functional ability of the family and freedom from pathology (Bradshaw, 1988). Duval and Miller (1985), from a developmental perspective, defined a healthy family as one that completes its developmental tasks at the appropriate time.

A holistic definition encompasses all aspects of family life, including interactions and health care functions. Public health and community welfare authors look at biostatistical indicators of family health. For example, these may include poverty rates, divorce rates, criminal and juvenile problems, high school dropout rates, and unemployment rates as indicators of family health. Family nursing authors may use nursing theory to define family health (i.e., Orem's self-care theory can refer to the extent to which the family assists its members in meeting their self-care requisites; Stanhope & Lancaster, 1996). It is clear that family health is more than the absence of disease or dysfunction; rather it is a state of well-being. In summary, family health is a dynamic, complex process that is affected by the family's cultural/ethnic heritage and various internal and external environmental factors. Table 5.1 provides examples of selected definitions.

FACTORS INFLUENCING FAMILY FUNCTIONING AND HEALTH

As discussed earlier, clinicians need a holistic, contextual view of the family in order to take advantage of opportunities for family-level change. This view

Table 5.1
Selected Definitions of Family Health

Family Health

- The family's quality of life as it is affected from a holistic perspective by such variables as nutrition, spirituality, environment, recreation, exercise, stress and coping, sexuality, health maintenance, and disease prevention (Bomar, 1989).

- The health of the individual members of the family as well as the health of the family unit as a whole.

- The dynamic process that includes the activities a family uses to promote and protect the well-being of the family as a unit and individual members.

- The process of expanding consciousness of the family. . . consciousness is defined as the informational capacity of the system and can be seen in the quantity and quality of interactions within the family and with the environment outside the family (Newman, 1983).

- Wellness and illness in interaction with the environment and five realms of the family experience: the interactive processes, the developmental processes, the coping processes, the integrity processes, and the health processes (K. Anderson and Tomlinson, 1992).

- The effectiveness of family functioning. It is a dynamic balance of family maintenance, family change, family togetherness, and individuation (Friedmann, 1989).

- Viewed as a distinction brought forth through relationships and languaging with other human beings and continually in interaction with a unique and changing environment (Wright, Watson, and Bell, 1990).

- As resilient to the ongoing events occurring between the family and its environment (McCubbin and McCubbin, 1993).

- A balance of cohesion and flexibility that is facilitated by good communication (Olson et al., 1986).

provides an opportunity to work with the family on many factors that influence family functioning and health. The Triangle of Family Health (see Figure 2.1) provides a context by which to understand both internal and external factors that can affect family functioning and health. These factors include physical health, psychological health, spiritual, environmental, and sociocultural conditions, and heredity (see Chapter 2 for discussion of each factor). Family structure and process factors also affect the family's ability to maintain its health. As these factors intertwine with each other, keeping all of the possibilities in mind will assist clinicians in working in the most constructive manner with the family.

FAMILY HEALTH PROMOTION

To be most helpful to families, clinicians must be concerned not only with the problems with which families present, but also with those activities that families participate in to promote their own family health. Health promotion is a major task of the family. When dialoging with families, clinicians will find a wide variance in health promotion activities among families, from none, to those keeping the family on the edge of health, to those that participate in many health promotion activities. The role of clinicians, when considering family health promotion, is to assist families in attaining, maintaining, and regaining the highest level of family health possible. This role involves clinicians taking up their education/teaching role when assisting families with health promotion.

In Danielson et al.'s (1993) Family Cycle of Health and Illness Model discussed in Chapter 3, family health promotion occurs in the first phase of the model. Family health promotion has been defined in several ways. Bomar (1996) defined family health promotion as family behaviors undertaken to increase the family's well-being or quality of life, whereas Pender's (1996) definition, which is somewhat similar, adds family activities that actualize the family's potentials. Family health promotion, however it is defined, involves the family's lifelong endeavors to nurture, care for, and empower the family and its members to reach their highest levels of health.

Although in the past, many health professionals focused mainly on individuals, dyads, or the community, it is imperative that clinicians focus on the *family unit* as this is where health behaviors, values, and beliefs are taught and learned. Family health promotion activities are important during both wellness and illness within the family unit. When one family member is experiencing an illness, the family must adapt to care for this member, while simultaneously allowing time and activities that promote health for all other family members.

The purpose of family health promotion activities is to strengthen the family as a unit. Pearsall (1990) in his book, *Power of the Family: Strength, Comfort, and Healing*, suggests ten strategies, to promote family health for lifelong family unity and caring. These ten strategies include the following:

1. Family rituals are the receptive behaviors or activities between two or more family members that occur with regularity in day-to-day activities. Examples are hugging when a member leaves or returns, saying grace at meals, and reading bedtime stories to children. Rituals provide security and attachment to oneness (unity) of the family system.

2. Family rhythm is learning to do things together. This is a calm moving together in harmony during the family activities of daily living.

3. Family reason is being reasonable during irrational times. Is there fairness and effort on everyone's part to reduce conflict? Recognize that family health is created not by being an actor but rather by interaction with others.

4. Family remembrance is keeping the family heritage, respecting family history, and learning from the conflicts of members from the previous generation.

5. Family resilience is the process of staying together through the stresses of life, to tolerate and grow as a unit with family spirit.

6. Family resonance is making good family "vibes." It is a sense of the family as a unit of energy, rather than as a group of individuals. Family members are free to self-actualize as well as to work together for family unity.

7. Family reconciliation is the process of getting back together again after conflict. This includes always forgiving, tolerating, and loving no matter what the family problem, as well as not allowing anything to destroy the family, because lack of forgiveness leads to a life of regret.

8. Family reverence is protecting the dignity of the family unit by concern for *us*. It means having a pride and respect for the uniqueness of the family unit and an enduring commitment to the eternal unity of the family.

9. Family revival is quick recovery from family conflicts, arguments, and feuds.

10. Family reunion is the process of assembling the family for the purpose of celebrating life together, maintaining family cohesion, comforting one another, learning from each other, and loving.

As clinicians with a systemic view dialogue with families, understanding how families stay healthy is as important as the problems that have brought the family to see the clinician. Clinicians can then use a combination of health promotion activities, as well as interventions for the presented problem, when working with families. With this approach, families can expand their resources for staying healthy and becoming healthier while dealing with the presenting problem.

ECOSYSTEM FACTORS INFLUENCING FAMILY HEALTH PROMOTION

Family health promotion is the outcome of the interaction and reciprocity between internal family system processes and external ecosystem factors that can affect the family's health promotion actions (Hanson, 2001; Hanson & Boyd, 1996). These factors are listed in Table 5.2 with comments for each.

Table 5.2
Factors Influencing Family Health Promotion

Internal Family System Factors	External Ecosystem Factors
Family type and development-flexible families are more likely to be involved in health promotion behaviors	National economy-affects availability of jobs, goods, and services for family needs; health promotion and disease prevention as priority in Healthy People 2010
Family structure-vulnerable families may spend less time on health promotion	Family economic resources-adequate income provides means for health promotion activities; vulnerable and poor families need assistance for better health
Family processes-functional communication passes on healthy values and beliefs about health promotion	Family policies-no specified national family policy; state and local governments administer family welfare programs
Culture/ethnicity-as these vary it is essential to assess cultural views about health promotion activities	Health policies-state, county, and city policies affect quality of family health; more collaboration needed among the many policymaking bodies for our diverse nation
Family lifestyle patterns-parents teach health patterns over the generations; one family member can effect change in the whole family	Environment-many public, occupational, and residential hazards; assist families in managing these
Religion-important factor in child, marital, and family health; provides support during transitions (weddings, confirmation), crisis, and loss; provides support groups	Media-visual and print media seldom target health promotion activities; recent media coverage of tobacco legislation and television advertisements concerning healthy parenting and drug use are examples of health promotion activities

Table 5.2.
Continued

Role models and change in role-family members role model health promotion behaviors both positive and negative	Cultural & societal norms-many diverse cultural/ethnic groups must intertwine with the society in which they live
Chronic illness-causes stress within the family and affects family's ability to engage in health promotion activities	Science and technology-more resources on family health promotion; advances have increased the number of family caregivers in the home and often compromises their health

Clinicians need to be positive role models related to family health promotion activities. They can discuss with the family how the family manages both the internal and external health promotion factors that relate to the problem that brought the family into treatment. For example, spirituality, often referred to as religion, has many positive affects on the family as it provides social support; encourages family togetherness through worship and family activities; provides a sense of meaning in life and for the family; promotes love, hope, faith, trust, forgiveness, goodness, self-control, morality, justice, and peace; encourages using spiritual assistance at times of family stress; and teaches reverence for family life (Hanson & Boyd, 1996). Clinicians can discuss with the family how they use this resource to help the family. Also, clinicians can discuss how other health promotion factors can assist families in dealing with their presenting problem. An evaluation can then be made to see how the family is implementing its health promotion activities.

QUESTIONS INQUIRING ABOUT FAMILY HEALTH AND FAMILY HEALTH PROMOTION

Clinicians must inquire about the health of each member of the family as well as the family as a unit. Paying attention to the cultural hierarchy will direct the clinician to whom to begin asking questions and the manner in which this should be done. For example, with Mexican-Americans, the clinician should address the father first and show respect and formality by using first and last names when introductions are made (Grothaus, 1996). As discussed in Chapter 3, during family interviews clinicians can pose four major types of questions—linear, circular, strategic, and reflexive (Tomm, 1987, 1988; Tomm & Lannamann, 1988). Table 3.5 gives examples of each of these types of questions. During various aspects of treatment, clinicians will frequently emphasize certain types of questions (Cox & Davis, 1993). When collecting information concerning the family's health and family health promotion activities, clinicians can use primarily linear questions to gather this type information. Clinicians might ask the following linear questions:

- When describing your family's health, what words would you use?
- Who in your family is the healthiest, next healthiest, and next?
- How often do members in your family see the family doctor?
- What is the health of family members outside of your household?
- What types of activities does your family do to stay healthy?
- How does your family work together in a healthy manner to solve problems?
- What does your family do together that you all really enjoy?
- What type of religious services do you attend as a family?

Clinicians also will want to know the outcomes of family health promotion activities related to the family's health. As much of this type of information is often gathered at the beginning of treatment, using circular questions at this time and to gather this information may lead to a higher level of therapeutic alliance between the clinician and family (Dozier et al., 1998; Ryan & Carr, 2001). The following types of circular questions can be used to explore the patterns between family health promotion activities and outcomes:

- When your family goes on vacation, how do you all get along?
- How does your family decide which movie to watch on TV?
- When the children get mad at each other, how do they resolve their problems?
- How do you see your religious values affecting the children?
- How do you all decide how to spend the holidays?

The information gathered from the family concerning health and health promotion activities can be placed on the family's genogram (see Chapter 6). Putting this information on the genogram will provide clinicians with a truly systemic visual representation of the family unit. This will assist clinicians in thinking and viewing the family systemically and will provide a context from which to understand the family and its presented problem.

QUESTIONS USED TO INQUIRE ABOUT INDIVIDUAL AND FAMILY ILLNESS/DISEASE

As clinicians can use linear and circular questions to understand family health and family health promotion, these same types of questions can be used to understand individual and family illness and disease. Although clinicians lacking medical background may not understand the physiological process and medical treatment of an illness or disease, they can understand the illness or disease from the family's perspective and the impact it has on individual and family functioning (Seaburn, 2001). Illness and disease have profound effects not only on the ill family member, but also on other individual family members and the family as a whole, both physically and mentally.

Additionally, it is important for clinicians to know about the existence of all illnesses and diseases within a family as medical and psychological disorders often have the same symptomology. Therefore, a family may believe that they are dealing with a mental disorder as the primary problem when in actuality, the mental disorder is secondary to a primary medical condition. Furthermore, it is possible that medications taken for a primary medical problem may have side effects that appear to be the symptoms of a major mental disorder. Therefore, clinicians first must rule out medical disorders before making a mental disorder diagnosis. On the other hand, it is possible for medical conditions and psychological problems to co-exist. In this case, there must be coordination of treatment for both conditions.

When using the multiaxial coding system of the *Diagnostic and Statistical Manual of Mental Disorders* (DSM-IV-TR; APA, 2000a), Axis III is used for the identification of physical disorders and conditions. It is only through identifying all of the problems that exist within a family that clinicians can provide the highest and most efficient and effective level of care. If medical and psychological problems do co-exist, clinicians must collaborate with other medical professionals to provide holistic care. This is especially true if medications are being taken for a medical condition and medications are being considered for treatment with a psychological condition simultaneously. It is possible that one medication can react adversely with other types of medication. Some medications have side effects that are the same as the disorder being treated. For example, an individual may be taking a medication for a medical problem that has the side effect of depression, while at the same time being treated for a primary mental disorder of depression. A high level of collaboration is necessary in such cases so that the individual receives the most effective treatment by both health professions.

The following are linear questions that clinicians can use to gather information about illnesses and diseases within a family:

• Who in your family has had health problems? What kind of problems were they?

• What kind of treatment has there been for the problem?

• What medical personnel are involved with you and your family?

• Did the treatment work or does the problem still exist?

• What kind of medications are being used for the problem?

• Have there been any problems when taking these medications?

- What difference did you notice after you started taking the medicine?
- Has your spirituality played a part in your dealing with this illness?

The following circular questions help clinicians to understand the patterns between illness and disease within a family and how the family is managing the problems:

- How has this problem affected you, your family, and your family life?
- How did you all manage when you found out there was no cure for the problem?
- What resources have been most helpful to you when dealing with this problem?
- As rehabilitation will take many months, how will the family deal with this?
- What medications did you find most or least helpful?
- How has your spirituality helped you find meaning in this situation?

Although treatment time allowed within the health care system is often short, clinicians must take the time to investigate all health factors that may be affecting the family. With thorough assessment of the family's health and illness, clinicians can then provide appropriate care. With permission of the client and family, clinicians can contact medical providers in order to provide care at the appropriate level of collaboration with other health professionals (Seaburn, 2001).

FAMILY HEALTH POLICY

The 1993 Family Leave Policy marked the beginning of an effort by the U.S. government to implement policies to improve the quality of family life and health. Family issues most often highlighted for debate by governmental bodies at the local, state, and national levels include marriage, divorce, abortion, child care, child health care, family violence, abuse, and family health insurance coverage. Decisions related to these issues should reflect the diversity of family structure, culture, and ethnicity. When working with individual families, clinicians must be aware of how these family issues might affect the families with whom they work. Although these may not be the presenting problem of the family, family health policy issues may play a direct or indirect part in the health of the family.

Having a wider public view, clinicians should be aware of and support policies that improve family health over the life span for all families. Wisensale (1993) suggested that family health policy should include: a national family policy agenda, universal access to health care, housing for low- and middle-income families, intergenerational family issues, and work and family issues (pp. 249–250). Clinicians can support and influence family policy legislation by doing the following:

1. Keeping informed about the issues

2. Communicating with legislators at all levels of government

3. Attending/speaking at hearings related to family policy issues

4. Becoming consultants to governmental committees

5. Belonging to a speakers union related to family health issues

6. Providing a health column in area newspapers

7. Giving expert testimony

8. Maintaining membership in and participating on committees in professional organizations

9. Supporting the political activities of professional organizations

SOCIAL POLICY AS A CONTEXT FOR LESBIAN AND GAY FAMILIES

All people live within the context of social policies that form their lives, mandate the opportunities available to them, and limit their capacity to succeed in a particular setting. Social policies establish rights and protections and delineate the rules and mutual responsibilities subsumed in both the unwritten and written social contracts between citizens and the state. The lesbian and gay men dyads, whether living as couples or in families, encounter a most complex and difficult relationship with the state and its various laws, rules, and procedures. These difficulties are experienced daily as lesbians and gay men live their lives.

Lesbians and gay men continue to be marginalized, discriminated against, unprotected, and even punished in our society. They are excluded from a variety of benefits and subjected to dramatic and subtle discriminatory policies and practices with very little opportunity for redress (Hartman, 1996). The field of family therapy has assumed heterosexuality in its very definition of family and has, generally, been silent on the entire subject of homosexuality. Every topic in the field gets discussed from a heterosexual perspective, except in those few instances in which gays and lesbians themselves have spoken or written about issues that pertain to their experiences (McGoldrick, 1996).

There have been recent attempts in the states of Hawaii (Marriage Project-Hawaii, 1999), California (McCarty, 1997), and Vermont (*Maranatha Christian Journal*, 2000) to pass legislation aimed at eliminating discrimination and the criminalization of same-sex sexual contact and to recognize formation of "legitimized" same-sex headed family units. Such legislative attempts have been attacked, vigorously, by conservatives, both fiscal and religious, under the guise that this type of legislation threatens the concept of *marriage*. Most of the legislation that has been passed has been carefully worded to refer to these units as civil unions in an effort to avoid furor of using the word, legitimizing the unions as marriages (Robinson, 2001). It is important to consider that most of the current legislation affecting lesbians, gay men, their children, and the families they form, is on the state level. This level of legislation is subject to scrutiny by the judicial branch of the federal government, the Supreme Court. There is, at present, no major federal legislation aimed at providing relief or benefits for lesbian and gay men's families.

Clinicians working with lesbian and gay men's families must keep in mind that social policy and social context must be considered within the clinician's treatment approach—as though social policy and context were living flesh-and-bone members of the family unit. These concepts and the pressures they exert are undeniable, unavoidable aspects of any lesbian or gay men's families.

Very often, liberal, straight clinicians underestimate the dangers and rejection faced by gay men and lesbians, pushing them to come out and characterizing their reluctance to do so as problematic, as internalized homophobia, and as pathological (Hartman, 1996). The clinician must incorporate a sense of time, place, circumstance, and cultural context when working with lesbian and gay men and their families. These families experience not only all of the problems and joys experienced by other families, but also must endure immense social, cultural, spirito-religious, and political pressures not imposed on other family groups.

COUNSELING POINTS

- Family health defined broadly and systemically provides the best context for care.
- Clinicians must assist families with health promotion activities to prevent problems.
- Clinicians must be aware of the internal family factors and ecosystem factors affecting family health promotion to provide the most assistance.
- Clinicians must inquire about all aspects of health and illness within the family.
- Family health policies, and the absence thereof, affect the health of families.
- Social policy can marginalize and discriminate against alternative family styles.

6

Family Assessment Tools

Ruth P. Cox, Norm Keltner, and Beverly Hogan

CULTURAL/HEALTH GENOGRAM

A genogram is a method of drawing a family tree that records information about the family, over at least three generations, to be used in assessment and treatment of the family (M. McGoldrick & Gerson, 1985). Bowen (1978) suggested that families repeat themselves in the same patterns from one generation to the next, including both psychosocial and health issues. Although McGoldrick and Gerson provided a standardized format and interpretive principles on which genograms are based, they also advised that theirs is only one way and "will no doubt be revised again in the future" (p. 1).

Indeed, the cultural/health genogram style suggested here is an expanded version of McGoldrick and Gerson's model in which the cultural heritage, spirituality, and health of the family are highlighted. The cultural/health genogram should be used in the assessment and treatment of the family, but is not to be confused with a type of cultural genogram suggested as a training tool to assist trainees (Hardy & Laszloffy, 1995). The purpose of Hardy and Laszloffy's type of genogram was to promote "cultural awareness and sensitivity by helping trainees to understand their cultural identities" (p. 228).

The cultural/health genogram (Figure 3.3) in this book provides clinicians with a graphic depiction of a family that maps information related to health and cultural heritage of the family over three generations, in addition to relational and systemic information about the family. The genogram of the Belcher family displays the basic skeleton of the three generation genogram along with many of the symbols that can be used to graphically describe a family (other standardized symbols can be found in McGoldrick & Gerson, 1985). Due to the amount of information displayed on this type of complex genogram, there are separate health and relationship legends to assist in understanding the symbols on the genogram. As family life will change over time, it is important to note that this genogram done at one point in time—1997—will appear differently when done at some future point in time.

For the cultural/health genogram, a variety of types of questions can be used to gather data during family interviews that will be useful to the family and clinician when solving family problems (see Section on interventive questions for family problem solving in Chapter 3). Although the clinician may not have a medical background, this should not dissuade questions and discussion of health and any medical problems (see earlier examples in Chapter 5). These types of questions can be useful during the assessment phase of work with families to broaden clinicians' view.

The genogram information gathered from the family initially can be done over several interviews, or one or two sessions can be devoted specifically to the genogram. M. McGoldrick and Gerson (1985) suggested an outline for the interview that includes gathering data from the family of origin, both sides of the family, ethnicity, major moves, significant others, and other information such as serious medical, behavioral, or emotional problems, job problems, drug/alcohol problems, legal problems, and other specific relational issues. Other information, such as spirituality or past solutions to problems, may be gathered depending on the clinician and the intended use of the genogram.

Accurately recording family data on the genogram is very important as the more knowledge clinicians have about the family over time, the more help they can be in assisting the family with their problem and attaining a higher level of wellness. Little empirical research has been done related to the accuracy in using the genogram as an assessment tool. However, some research has shown that clinicians are more accurate about recording some data (i.e., names and symbols), moderately accurate in recording unnamed persons, relationship descriptors, medical issues, personal issues, descriptive phases, and most inaccurate in recording other data (i.e., dates and ages; Coupland, Serovich, & Glenn, 1995). Therefore, clinicians should be very attentive when using this expanded cultural/health genogram model to allow this tool to be of the greatest help to clinicians and families when working on family problems.

Family culture, ethnicity, and health make up the context in which relationships, both within and outside the family, are developed over time. Access to this type of information will inform clinicians as they work with the family toward a higher level of wellness and health. Descriptors of types of relationships within the family, such as very close, close, cut off, distant, and conflictual, are drawn on the genogram and the meaning of each can be found in the relationship legend. Information on the cultural/health genogram for each family member (when known) and where the symbol for the information can be found are as follows:

- Cultural heritage (identified within the genogram structure)

- Religious/spiritual affiliation (identified within the genogram structure)

- Health (health legend)

- Illness with identified problem (health legend)

- Pets or other significant animals within the family system (relationship legend)
- Affiliations outside the family unit (relationship legend)
- Relationships within and outside the family unit (relationship legend)
- Relationships valued but not of biological origin (relationship legend)
- Profession or occupation (identified within the genogram structure)
- Critical events affecting the family unit and system (on the genogram or listed separately)

Interpreting genograms for clinical use can involve different categories as suggested by M. McGoldrick and Gerson (1985). Although using these types of categories is one example of how to use genograms, these authors stated there are inexhaustible factors that can be considered in interpreting genograms. For example, DeMaria, Weeks, and Hof (1999) suggested the use of focused genograms that explore one aspect of the family, such as attachments, emotions, gender, sexuality and romantic love. Kuehl (1995) suggested the genogram can be used "to include the basic tenets and techniques of solution-oriented therapies" (p. 239). Like these authors, the factors suggested in this book for the cultural/health genogram are some of many ways to make genograms clinically useful. However, this type of genogram includes, in one drawing, all the spheres of impact that can affect a family, making it more useful to clinicians.

Clinically relevant working hypotheses about family patterns can be generated from the following categories (M. McGoldrick & Gerson, 1985, pp. 39–124). After each category are some ideas that may be helpful in generating hypotheses:

Category 1: Family Structure

Household composition
Sibling constellation
Unusual family configurations

Generating hypotheses: "By examining the family structure alone one can hypothesize about certain themes, roles, and relationships which may then be checked out by eliciting further information about the family" (p. 70).

Category 2: Life-Cycle Fit

Normative time expectations for each phase of the family life cycle
Time between meeting, engagement and marriage, and dissolution of marriage
Life-cycle discrepancies

Generating hypotheses: "In sum, ages and dates on the genogram allow one to see what life cycle transitions the family is adapting to and whether life cycle events and ages occur within normative expectations. When they do not, possible difficulties in managing that phase of the life cycle can be further explored" (p. 74).

Category 3: Pattern Repetition Across Generations

Patterns of functioning

Patterns of relationships

Repeated structural patterns

Generating hypotheses: "To summarize the principle for interpreting pattern repetition across generations, repetitive patterns of functioning, relationships, and family structure on a genogram suggest the possibility of the patterns continuing in the present and into the future. Recognition of these patterns offers the possibility of helping family members alter these patterns" (p. 83).

Category 4: Life Events and Family Functioning

The coincidences of life events

The impact of life changes, transitions, and traumas

Anniversary reactions

Social, economic, and political events

Generating hypotheses: "In sum, tracking critical events and changes in family functioning allows us to make systemic connections between seeming coincidences, assess the impact of traumatic changes on family functioning and its vulnerability to future stresses, track anniversary reactions, and then try to understand such events in the larger social, economic and political context" (p. 96).

Category 5: Relational Patterns and Triangles

Triangles

Parent–child triangles

Common couple triangles

Triangles in divorced and remarried families

Triangles in families with foster or adopted children

Multigenerational triangles

Relationships outside the family

Generating hypotheses: "In sum, the genogram allows the clinician to detect intense relationships in a family and, given the family's structure and position in the life cycle, to hypothesize about the important triangular patterns and boundaries of that family. Understanding such triangular patterns is essential in planning clinical interventions. 'Detriangling' is an important clinical process through which family members are coached to free themselves from rigid triangular patterns" (p. 114).

Category 6: Family Balance and Imbalance—Functional Whole of a Family System

The family structure

Roles

Level and style of functioning

Resources

Generating hypotheses: "In sum, reading the genogram for patterns of contrast and balance in the family structure, roles, functioning, and resources allows the clinician to derive hypotheses about how the family is adapting to imbalances that may be stressing the system" (p. 124).

These categories can be used with the cultural/health genogram found in this book. However, to be most useful, the use of these categories and hypotheses must be *embedded* within the family context of culture, health, and spirituality in order for clinicians to have the broadest understanding of the family and to be the most helpful to the family. Questions used in gaining the information in these categories must be asked within the context of the family's culture and the effects of this culture on the family over past generations and in the present. Clinicians must assess the family's spirituality and its pervasive effects from the past, the present, and into the future while simultaneously using these categories. Data concerning the family and individual health over generations and how families have dealt with illness in the past will widen clinicians' view of the family's problem-solving skills.

Genograms can be used clinically in a variety of ways (M. McGoldrick & Gerson, 1985). Some of the uses are "to engage the whole family, to unblock the system, to clarify family patterns, and to reframe and detoxify family issues" (p. 125). Other examples of genograms use include record-keeping, designing strategic interventions, use as a quasi-projective technique (Wachtel, 1982), and designing solution-oriented interventions (Kuehl, 1995). In a health care family practice, genograms can be used for systemic medical record-keeping, rapport-building, and medical management and preventive medicine (M. McGoldrick & Gerson, 1985). Although these are only examples, the genogram is a tool that can be used in a variety of ways, in a variety of settings, when working with families. The case study at the end of the book illustrates the use of a genogram.

ECOMAP

The ecomap is a visual representation of the family and it linkages to its larger social system (e.g., friends, jobs, spiritual/religious organization, schools, social service agencies, community organizations, recreational activities, health care system, legal system, and volunteer organizations). According to B. Ross and Cobb (1990), the ecomap is "an overview of the family in their situation, picturing both the important nurturant and stress-producing connections between the family and the world" (p. 176). Like genograms, information for the ecomap can be gathered from the family initially over several interviews with the family or one or two sessions can be devoted specifically to the ecomap. Ecomaps can be updated as changes occur within the family system.

Family culture, ethnicity, and health make up the context in which relationships outside the family are developed over time. The ecomap provides an integrated, more specific view of the family situation within its larger context. Whereas a genogram identifies relationships outside the family that affect the family, the ecomap specifically identifies the exchange of energy and resources between and among these relationships. For clinicians, this provides more information about family patterns as they interact within the larger social system. This larger social system may include the local environment and/or interactions at the state, regional, national, and international level. When there are problems within the family that involve relationships in this larger environment, these relationships may play a significant role in family functioning and well-being. In this case, clinicians may call on these significant others in the family network to play a part in the solution to the current family problems. As various social agencies may direct the family differently from the clinician, collaboration among all those interested in the family will allow for co-construction of workable solutions for the present predicaments that will lead to a higher level of well-being for the family (H. Anderson & Goolishian, 1988).

Figure 6.1 illustrates an ecomap of the Belcher family. It starts with a large circle with the family genogram in the center and with smaller circles outside representing "significant persons, agencies, and institutions in the family's context" (Wright & Leahey, 1994, p. 56). Lines are drawn between the outside circles and the family members to depict the nature of the relationship (see legend in Figure 6.1). Arrows are used to show the flow of energy and resources between people and between the family and the outside environment.

Interpreting ecomaps for clinical use will involve different external factors within the suprasystem for each family that are specific to that family situation. The family's cultural heritage and values must be considered when identifying suprasystem linkages as different cultures direct families in how they interact with the world. Working in this way, clinicians will not overlook powerful significant other relationships that can assist the family with their problems. This will allow clinicians to work with those who have influence with the family and the problem to ensure they are working with those who have the power to make changes. Such a view allows for more effectiveness as the larger macrosystem is taken into account when working with the family. Categories for these factors include significant others, agencies, and institutions. Although

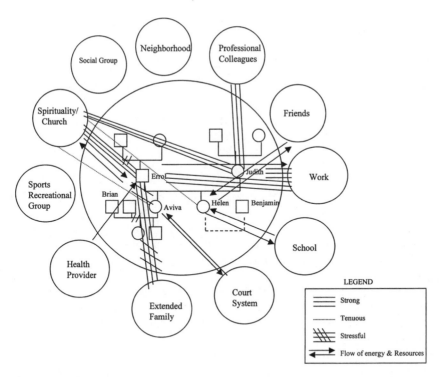

Figure 6.1. Ecomap.

using these types of factors is one example of how to use ecomaps, there are inexhaustible factors that can be considered in interpreting ecomaps.

Clinically relevant working hypotheses about family patterns can be generated from viewing the suprasystem persons, agencies, and institutions that have relationships with the family. These hypotheses can include the following:

Category 1: Significant others

Generating hypotheses: By examining those with whom the family has relationships within the suprasystem, one can hypothesize about certain themes and roles that may then be checked out by eliciting more information about the family.

Category 2: Agencies

Generating hypotheses: By examining events and changes in the family necessitating systemic connections with community agencies, clinicians can hypothesize about the family events and the use or non-use of larger social and economic agencies.

Category 3: Institutions

Generating hypotheses: Reading the ecomap for patterns of balance in the family structure, roles, functioning, and suprasystem resources allows clinicians to derive hypotheses about how the family is adapting to imbalances that may be stressing the family system.

These categories for the ecomap can be used in conjunction with the cultural/health genogram to provide clinicians with a broader perspective, a metaview of the family within in system context. To be most useful, the use of these categories and hypotheses must be embedded within the family context of culture, health, and spirituality for clinicians to have the broadest suprasystem understanding of the family. Questions used in gaining the information in these categories must be asked within the context of the family's culture and the effects of this culture on the family over past generations and in the present. Clinicians must assess the family's spirituality and its pervasive effects from the past, the present, and into the future while simultaneously using these categories. Data concerning the family and individual health over the generations and how families have dealt with illness in the past will widen the clinician's view of the family's relationships with the suprasystem in which it resides.

Ecomaps can be used clinically in a variety of ways (Hanson, 2001; Hanson & Boyd, 1996). Some of these uses are to establish rapport between clinician and family, to organize many facts, to set goals in intervention in and of itself, and as a teaching tool.

Other uses include discussion with the family concerning resources available in the community and deciding which of these resources the family has and might want to use, increasing clinician awareness of the family within its community, and assisting in the assessment and planning phase of treatment (Swanson & Niles, 1997). Although these are only examples, the ecomap is a tool that can be used in a variety of ways, in a variety of settings, when working with families. The case study at the end of the book illustrates the use of an ecomap along with a genogram.

FAMILY HEALTH AND FUNCTIONING ASSESSMENT

A family assessment guideline can assist in "thinking family systems" (see Table 6.1). It uses theory to direct data gathering concerning family interactions, explores family knowledge of health and illness, identifies desired family goals, and indicates family-level interventions. Through dialogues based on a guide, families can be actively engaged in decision making regarding self-health priorities (Lapp, Diemert, & Enestvedt, 1993). "The family perspective serves to expand the scope of practice, to increase insight, to allow for case finding, and to move health intervention to a more holistic dimension" (p. 310). Theoretical/conceptual perspectives incorporated into this family assessment include family systems theory (Bowen, 1978), Circumplex Model (Olson et al., 1985), cultural heritage (Giger & Davidhizar, 1995), health and health promotion, and cultural/health genograms (M. McGoldrick & Gerson, 1985).

Table 6.1.
Guideline for Family Health and Functioning Assessment

I. Interview family and obtain the following data:

    A. Demographic and family composition:

        1. Complete a Three-Generation Genogram including:

            a. pets if applicable

            b. the cultural heritage of all family members

            c. the health status of each family member (Legend)

        2. Complete a Ecomap of the Family

    B. Family Interactions

        Identify, discuss, and give examples for each of the following:

        1. Family Structure

            a. Subsystems-identify all five subsystems

            b. Boundaries-include internal and external

            c. Roles of each family member

            d. Rules of the family - procedural and relational

            e. Triangles-identify all triangles (specify parentification and/or

               scapegoating)

        2. Family Process

            a. Separateness/Connectedness-describe this including sexuality

            b. Enmeshment/Disengagement-classify the family by one of these

            c. Communication-who communicates with whom and how

            d. Power-identify who has the power in the family

            e. Secrets/Myths-how does this effect family process?

        3. Family Spirituality

            a. Method by which family members expresses their spirituality

    C. Family Relationship Map

        1. Identify the family type according to Olson and any family concerns

**Table 6.1.
Continued**

II. Cultural Aspects

   Describe how each of the cultural variables are operationalized within the family:

   A. Time

   B. Space

   C. Communication

   D. Social organization

   E. Biological variations

   F. Environmental control

III. Summary

   A. Discuss individual developmental and health problems in relationship to family

      structure, family process, family spirituality, and health.

   Discuss the family using the traits of a healthy family.

   B. Discuss family strengths related to structure, process, spirituality, and health.

   C. Discuss family problems related to structure, process, spirituality, and health.

   D. Discuss the family's response to the interview. Discuss external and internal factors

      that influence the family's health promotion.

IV. Goals/Interventions

   Indicate family goals and plans for interventions and/or referrals with justification from

      Categories I, II,and III.

Families and health are woven together. Therefore, assessment also includes the health problems of each family member and those that may be a result of dealing with family problems. Greenberg et al. (1993) found that caregivers' subjective burdens related to stigma and worry were significant predictors of negative physical health. As families cope in different ways, assessment of family-coping methods will provide valuable data when discussing interventions with the family.

The family assessment model shown in Table 6.1 starts with a genogram and has three assessment categories for Family Interactions with subcategories:

structural, process, and spiritual. The clinician then identifies the family type according to the Olson model. The second major section of the family assessional deals with cultural aspects of the family life. Operationalized in the model are those concepts of a healthy family, health promotion, and family stages, viewed through the lens of culture within the larger system in which the family resides (see Figure 4.2). The case study at the end of the book illustrates the use of an assessment with the Belcher family.

MEDICATIONS COMMONLY USED WITH MENTAL HEALTH PROBLEMS

Current thinking, when considering the brain's chemistry and mental disorders, proposes a direct relation between psychiatric/emotional disorders and altered brain chemistry. Although the direction of influence probably flows from chemical changes to cognitive/emotional/behavioral symptoms, some suggest a reversal of this cause and effect hypothesis (i.e., symptoms and experiences change brain chemistries). Whatever future discoveries may reveal in this regard, clients in need of mental health services tend to have biochemical irregularities. Psychiatric drugs work by modifying those irregularities. Specifically, most psychiatric drugs exert their effect by manipulating neurotransmitters and neurotransmitter systems.

Neurotransmitters

Normal brain function depends on normal neurotransmitter function. Scientists identify more than fifty neurotransmitters, however, knowledge of only five of the neurotransmitters gives the health clinician enough information to effectively work with clients. Neurotransmitters of significance include norepinephrine, serotonin, dopamine, acetylcholine, and gamma amino butyric acid (GABA) (Keltner, 2000a; Keltner, Hogan, & Guy, 2001; Keltner, Hogan, Knight, & Royals, in press). Each of these neurotransmitters affects brain areas implicated in mental disorders. Furthermore, commonly used psychiatric drugs typically affect one or more of these five neurotransmitters. By having a modest understanding of these neurotransmitters, clinicians can effectively respond to clients and families in many cases. Table 6.2 provides a simplistic, but accurate depiction of the role of neurotransmitters in common psychiatric disorders.

Psychiatric Drugs

Psychiatric drugs (i.e., psychotropic drugs, psychopharmacologic agents) work in most cases on neurotransmitter systems. This section focuses on the basic categories of these drugs. Taking our lead from Table 6.2, discussion of antidepressants, antimanic, antianxiety, antipsychotic, and antidementia drugs follows. A table following each section lists commonly used psychiatric drugs with both generic and trade names, daily adult dosages, and side effects.

Table 6.2.
Role of Neurotransmitters in Common Mental Health/Psychiatric Disorders

Neurotransmitter	Deficiency/ Elevation	Mental Health Disorder
Norepinephrine	Deficiency	Depression
Norepinephrine	Elevation	Anxiety, mania
Serotonin	Deficiency	Depression
Serotonin	Elevation	Anxiety, sexual dysfunction
Dopamine	Deficiency	Movement disorders, sexual dysfunction
Dopamine	Elevation	Schizophrenia, psychotic thinking
Acetylcholine	Deficiency	Memory problems, Alzheimer's disease
GABA	Deficiency	Anxiety

Antidepressant Drugs

Antidepressant drugs work on increasing the deficiencies in norepinephrine and/or serotonin noted in Table 6.2 (Keltner, 2000b; Stahl, 1998). Some drugs fall easily into drug categories because of similarities in chemical structure or mechanisms of action (i.e., how they work). A few newer drugs defy categorization and stand alone. Drugs easily categorized lead the discussion.

Tricyclic antidepressants (TCAs) include familiar drugs such as Elavil and Pamelor. TCAs elevate both norepinephrine and serotonin. TCA effectiveness, although well established, yields to disturbing and potentially serious side effects. Newer drugs, although no more effective than TCAs, often achieve higher prescription rates related to better side-effect profiles. Side effects of particular concern for TCAs include effects on memory (i.e., anticholinergic effect), effects on blood pressure (i.e., antiadrenergic effect), and effects on heart function (Keltner & Folks, 2001). Furthermore, TCAs possess a narrow therapeutic index that simply highlights the similarity between the dose needed to help someone versus the dose needed to kill someone.

Selective serotonin reuptake inhibitors (SSRIs) include drugs such as Prozac, Paxil, Zoloft, and Celexa. Referring to Table 6.2, one notes that an antidepressant probably acts on norepinephrine, serotonin, or both (Keltner & Folks, 2001). As their name suggests, SSRIs selectively increase serotonin. SSRIs, although relatively safe drugs, have two side effects of concern. First, a significant number of clients lose their interest and ability to engage in sexual activity.

Second, many clients suffer gastrointestinal effects such as nausea, vomiting, and diarrhea.

Novel antidepressants, not easily categorized, include Effexor, Wellbutrin, Serzone, and Remeron. In one way or the other, each of these drugs boost serotonin and/or norepinephrine. The exception is Wellbutrin, which also causes an increase in dopamine. This particular chemical attribute of Wellbutrin makes it (under the trade name Zyban) useful in smoking-cessation programs (Keltner & Folks, 2001).

Monoamine oxidase inhibitors (MAOIs) include drugs such as Nardil and Parnate. Because of severe side effects and potentially lethal drug–drug or food–drug interactions, few physicians prescribe these agents. Labels on many over-the-counter (OTC) drugs include warnings to avoid mixing that particular drug with an MAOI. Some OTC preparations, when combined with an MAOI, have proven lethal. A newer, more specialized MAOI, moclobemide, does not carry this same level of risk (Keltner & Folks, 2001).

Antimanic Drugs (Mood Stabilizers)

Antimanic drugs or mood stabilizers normalize brain activity. Clients experiencing manic episodes endure emotional, cognitive, and behavioral upheaval including racing thoughts, hyperactivity, annoying and frightening intrusive behaviors, euphoria, elevated and/or irritable mood, and swings in temperament. Three types of antimanic agents benefit these clients—lithium, certain anticonvulsants, and an atypical antipsychotic.

Lithium, a naturally occurring element, stabilizes mood by substituting for sodium, a chemical needed for brain-cell activity. By substituting for sodium, lithium slows down brain activity (Keltner & Folks, 2001). Lithium, as do TCAs, has a narrow therapeutic index meaning only a slight difference exists between a therapeutic dose and a toxic or even lethal dose. Hence, lithium blood-level monitoring must occur frequently (normal = 0.6 to 1.2 mEq/liters; toxicity develops over 1.5 mEq/liters). Common side effects of lithium include fine tremor, nausea, polydipsia (excessive drinking), and polyuria (excessive urination). Gross tremor, slurred speech, or cognitive changes indicate toxicity and should trigger a call to the prescriber.

Two anticonvulsives, Depakene and Tegretol, decrease symptoms of mania. Although working via other mechanisms, these drugs slow down and normalize brain activity as well. Serious side effects seldom occur with Depakene, but Tegretol may cause serious blood abnormalities. More common effects associated with Tegretol include drowsiness and dizziness.

Olanzapine (Zyprexa), an atypical antipsychotic agent, has been recently approved for the treatment of bipolar disorder (Keltner, Coffeen, & Johnson, 2000; Keltner & Folks, 2001). It has proven effective and adds to the arsenal of drugs available for this devastating condition. Olanzapine is discussed in the antipsychotic section as well.

Table 6.3.
Commonly Used Antidepressants

Antidepressant Drugs	Daily Adult Dosage (mg/day)	Side Effects
TCAs		*Anticholinergic*
amitriptyline (Elavil)	75–300	Dry mouth, blurred vision, constipation, urinary hesitancy
clomipramine (Anafranil)	75–200	*Antiadrenergic*
desipramine (Norpramin)	75–300	Orthostatic hypotension (B/P drops upon rising)
doxepin (Sinequan)	75–300	*Cardiac*
imipramine (Tofranil)	75–300	Arrthymias, palpitations, tachycardia
nortriptyline (Pamelor)	50–200	
SSRIs		*Central Nervous System*
citalopram (Celexa)	10–60	Dizziness, tremor, insomnia, somnolence, agitation
fluoxetine (Prozac)	10–80	*Anticholinergic*
paroxetine (Paxil)	10–60	Dry mouth, constipation, diarrhea, gas
sertraline (Zoloft)	25–200	*Other*
		Sexual dysfunction, nausea, vomiting
Novel Antidepressants		
		Bupropion—risk of seizures at high doses, dry mouth, insomnia
bupropion (Wellbutrin)	150–450	*Mirtazapine*—somnolence, increased appetite, weight gain, dizziness, increase in cholesterol
mirtazapine (Remeron)	20–35	*Nefazodone*—headache, somnolence, dizziness, insomnia, light headedness, dry mouth nausea, constipation
nefazodone (Serzone)	100–600	*Venlafaxine*—headache, somnolence, dizziness, insomnia, nervousness, nausea, dry mouth, constipation, abnormal orgasm
venlafaxine (Effexor)	150–450	

Source: Adapted from: Keltner and Folks (2001).

Table 6.4.
Commonly Used Antimanic (or Mood Stabilizing) Drugs

Antimanic Drugs	Daily Adult Dosage (mg/day)	Side Effects
lithium (Eskalith, Lithane, Lithobid, others)	900–1200	Fine tremor, nausea, polydipsia, polyruria
Anticonvulsants		
valproates — (Depakene, Depakote)	750–1500	*Valproates*—transient hair loss, weight gain, tremors, GI upset, pancreatitis
carbamazepine (Tegretol)	800–1200	*Carbamazepine*—skin reactions, blood dyscrasias, sedation, poor coordination, hyponatremia
Antipsychotics		
Olanzapine (Zyprexa)	15–45	Insomnia, sedation, weight gain, dry mouth, constipation, sexual dysfunction

Source: Adapted from Keltner and Folks (2001).

Antianxiety Drugs

Benzodiazepine antianxiety drugs or anxiolytics include drugs from the benzodiazepine family (i.e., Valium, Ativan, Xanax, and Librium). The benzodiazepine drugs work by affecting the GABA system (see Table 6.2). When stimulated, the GABA system slows down brain-cell firing. Benzodiazepines cause a pleasant subdued experience, thus they appeal to individuals seeking such a sensation. Abuse of benzodiazepines occurs commonly. Medicinal drugs that depress the central nervous system add to the effects of benzodiazepines as do drugs used for recreational purposes (e.g., alcohol and other "downers"). Although safe alone, benzodiazepines coupled with other depressants have resulted in deaths (Keltner & Folks, 2001). The technical explanation as to why benzodiazepines (alone) do not cause death in overdose, but can cause death when combined with other drugs, goes beyond the scope of this text (see Lehne, 2001, for a discussion of this issue).

A nonbenzodiazepine drug, BuSpar, possesses several advantages and disadvantages compared to the benzodiazepines. First, it does not cause the same psychological effects as the benzodiazepines, thus it does not pose an abuse potential. Second, BuSpar precipitates few drug interactions. For example,

BuSpar combined with alcohol theoretically should not trigger a reaction. Disadvantages of BuSpar include a significant delay between initiating treatment and symptom relief from anxiety. Up to six weeks can pass before a therapeutic or optimal response develops. The precise mechanism by which BuSpar generates an antianxiety effect remains unknown.

Antipsychotic Drugs

Antipsychotics (also know as neuroleptics, major tranquilizers) include traditional agents such as Haldol, Thorazine, and Stelazine, and newer atypical agents such as Clozaril, Zyprexa, and Risperdal. All of these drugs work by blocking receptors to which dopamine attaches (see Table 6.2 indicating the relation between schizophrenia and elevated dopamine levels; Keltner, Hogan, & Guy, 2001). Other mechanisms also account for antipsychotic effectiveness but the intricacies of those mechanisms lie outside the basic objectives of this text. Important distinctions between traditional and atypical antipsychotics warrant mention.

Traditional antipsychotics, although considerably less expensive, have slipped in popularity because of three categories of significant side effects; anticholinergic effects, antiadrenergic effects, and extrapyramidal side effects (EPSEs or EPS). A review of these side effects follows this section.

Table 6.5.
Commonly Used Antianxiety Drugs

Antianxiety Drugs	Daily Adult Dosage (mg/day)	Side Effects
Benzodiazepines		
alprazolam (Xanax)	0.75–4	Oversedation, memory
lorazepam (Ativan)	2–6	impairment, paradoxical
oxazepam (Serax)	30–60	excitement, emotional blunting,
chlordiazepoxide (Librium)	15–100	depression, drowsiness, fatigue, mental impairment
clonazepam (Klonopin)	0.5–10	
diazepam (Valium)	4–40	
Nonbenzodiazepine		Dizziness, headache, depression,
buspirone (BuSpar)	15–40	stimulation, insomnia, nervousness, lightheadedness tremors, dry mouth, constipation

Source: Adapted from Keltner and Folks (2001).

Atypical antipsychotic drugs produce fewer of these annoying and dangerous side effects plus attack symptoms not affected by traditional agents (the so-called negative symptoms). Although not causing as many EPSEs as traditional drugs, atypical agents do cause significant weight gain (at least one client gained sixty pounds on Zyprexa). Furthermore, Clozaril may induce a condition referred to as agranulocytosis, a steep and potentially fatal drop in white blood cells. Because of the risk of overwhelming infection, the manufacturer of Clozaril requires weekly or biweekly blood specimens to monitor white blood cell levels (Keltner, et al., 2000).

As noted eacher, atypical antipsychotics cost considerably more than do traditional drugs. For example, a month's supply of Haldol may be purchased for $20 or less, whereas a month's supply of Zyprexa may cost $300 to $400. As in many cases, the expense of atypical drugs creates a prohibitive barrier for some individuals.

Antidementia Drugs (Drugs for Alzheimer's Disease)

Cholinesterase inhibitor antidementia drugs (drugs for Alzheimer's disease) include Cognex, Aricept, and the newer agent, Exelon. Referring to Table 6.2, note that a deficiency in the neurotransmitter acetylcholine contributes to Alzheimer's disease. The use of the term *contributes* correctly suggests that acetylcholine deficiency provides only a partial explanation. Although discussing other brain pathologies would enhance one's understanding of Alzheimer's disease, the most effective treatments manipulate acetylcholine levels, hence our concentration on these drugs (Keltner, Zielinski, & Hardin, 2001). All three drugs work by preventing the natural breakdown of acetylcholine. All neurotransmitters have a life cycle that includes their birth (i.e., synthesis) and their change to another chemical (i.e., metabolism). Because acetylcholine exists in lower than normal quantities in clients with Alzheimer's disease, blocking its metabolism increases its functional availability. Cognex, due to liver toxicities, no longer captures much of the market. Aricept and Exelon cause few significant side effects, although manufacturers' reports acknowledge common occurrence of gastrointestinal and some central nervous effects (e.g., insomnia, headache, dizziness).

Side Effects of Psychiatric Drugs

Psychiatric drugs cause side effects too numerous to review in such a brief text. However, three categories of side effects worth noting are anticholinergic, antiadrenergic, and extrapyramidal side effects. These types of side effects occur as a reaction to many psychiatric drugs, so their review merits comment.

Anticholinergic Side Effects

Anticholinergic effects develop due to blockage of the acetylcholine neurotransmitter system. Anyone who has ever taken a Benadryl tablet has expe-

Table 6.6.
Commonly Used Antipsychotic Drugs

Antipsychotic Drugs	Daily Adult Dosage (mg/day)	Side Effects
Traditional		
chlorpromazine (Thorazine)	30–800	Extrapyramidal side effects (EPSEs)
fluphenazine (Prolixin)	0.5–20	Anticholinergic effects
haloperidol (Haldol)	1–15	Antiadrenergic effects
loxapine (Loxitane)	20–250	Endocrine effects: enlarged breast, lactation
thioridazine (Mellaril)	150–800	Cardiac effects: can cause arrhymthias
Atypical		
clozapine (Clozaril)	300–900	*Most atypicals* can cause weight gain, low to high levels of sedation, orthostasis, and anticholinergic effects.
olanzapine (Zyprexa)	5–40	
quetiapine (Seroquel)	300–400	
risperidone (Risperdal)	4–16	*Clozapine* is known to cause a potentially fatal condition known as agranulocytosis. Clozapine can also cause excessive drooling.
ziprasidone (Geodon)	80–160	
		Ziprasidone is thought to not cause significant weight gain.

Source: Adapted from Keltner and Folks (2001).

rienced anticholinergic side effects, such as dry mouth, dried up nasal passages, and constipating tendencies. Other anticholinergic effects may or may not include blurred vision (the optometrist uses anticholinergic eye drops to dilate pupils), decreased sweating, increased heart rate, and difficulty starting a stream of urine (Keltner, 2000a; Keltner, Hogan, Knight, & Royals, in press). A decrease in availability of acetylcholine leads to memory problems as well (Table 6.2). Beyond the dry mouth, and so on, memory difficulties and confused thinking develop as significant effects of drugs with anticholinergic properties and susceptibility increases in older individuals. TCAs and other highly anticholinergic drugs can cause pronounced cognitive dysfunction.

Sometimes side effects of antipsychotic drugs require the co-administration of an anticholinergic drug. Cogentin can offset many of the extrapyramidal

Table 6.7.
Commonly Used Drugs for Dementia

Antidementia Drugs	Daily Adult Dosage (mg/day)	Side Effects
Cholinesterase inhibitors		GI upset, insomnia, headache, dizziness, irritability, aggression, increased libido
donepezil (Aricept)	5–10	
rivastigmine (Exelon)	6–12	*Tacrine* is known to cause significant liver toxicity.
tacrine (Cognex)	40–160	

Source: Adapted from Keltner and Folks (2001).

side effects of most antipsychotics. However, Cogentin worsens the EPSE tardive dyskinesia.

Antiadrenergic Side Effects

Antiadrenergic side effects typically result from blockage of certain receptors on blood vessels. Normally, these receptors cause blood vessel constriction, for instance when one stands. When this function becomes compromised, blood vessels dilate instead of constricting, thus allowing a pooling of blood in the legs. When this occurs, people become lightheaded and may pass out. Many injuries result from antiadrenergic effects.

Extrapyramidal Side Effects

Extrapyramidal side effects develop as a result of decreased levels of dopamine, which upsets the natural balance in certain parts of the brain between dopamine, and acetylcholine (note how the same neurotransmitters keep coming up). Note that too much dopamine contributes to schizophrenia and psychosis, whereas too little dopamine causes movement disorders (e.g., Parkinson's disease). Drugs used in the treatment of schizophrenia have in common their ability to block dopamine receptors (Keltner, Hogan, & Guy, 2001). In so doing, these agents often create drug-induced movement disorders. Specific EPSEs include akathisia, the irresistible urge to move; akinesia, the inability to move; dystonia, the sustained/twisted contraction of a muscle group (e.g., the neck); Parkinsonism, rigidity, tremor, bradykinesia; tardive dyskinesia late onset, squirming movements of mouth, tongue, or other body parts.

Treatment of EPSEs typically includes a drug that blocks acetylcholine receptors (i.e., an anticholinergic) such as Cogentin. The technical explanation for this exception lies outside the scope of this text.

Interactions Between Psychiatric Drugs and Other Drugs

Many interactions between psychiatric agents and other drugs could be listed. Rather than attempt to enumerate all of those interactions, a discussion of three general interaction principles follows.

Additive Effects

Additive effects result with the co-administration of drugs with similar properties. For example, an additive effect develops when combining Valium (a central nervous system depressant) and alcohol (a central nervous system depressant).

Enzyme Induction or Inhibition

Most drugs and all neurotransmitters change as a result of enzyme activity. If enzyme activity increases (i.e., enzyme induction), then substrates of that enzyme change more rapidly, hence that drug tends to have less effect (Keltner, Schwecke, & Bostrom, in press). If, on the other hand, enzyme activity slows down (i.e., enzyme inhibition), the drugs metabolized by that enzyme tend to have greater effect (because the drug remains intact longer). Decreased drug effect leads to potential symptom breakthrough (less drug equals more symptom potential). Increased drug effect leads to potential for drug toxicity (more drug equals toxic effect potential). Although enzyme induction or inhibition embraces complex concepts, this covers the basics.

Competition for Protein Binding

Another mechanism of drug interaction concerns the binding of psychiatric drugs to blood or plasma proteins. Most drugs bind to blood proteins in some fixed ratio. For example, about 98% of Elavil binds to proteins (Keltner, Schwecke, & Bostrom, in press). It does not matter whether the client takes 25 mg or 100 mg—98% of the Elavil in circulation will bind to proteins. Drug molecules bound to protein do not cause an effect. So, in the case of Elavil, only 2% of the drug creates an antidepressant effect. Drug interactions can occur when two drugs, both highly attracted to plasma proteins, compete for binding sites. If, for example, Elavil binding drops from 98% to 96%, then 4% becomes active. This doubles the amount of Elavil affecting the brain (from 2% to 4%) for a 100% increase in active drug. Competition for protein-binding sites contributes to drug interactions.

Psychiatric Medications: Concerns for Clinicians

The nonmedically trained, licensed clinician does not have direct legal responsibility for monitoring medications, though it is an issue impacting client care and responses to counseling. There are three primary concerns of the clinician when working with a client on psychiatric medications: side effects, safety, and attitudes toward medication.

Side Effects

Clients see their clinicians more frequently than their physicians, so despite the fact that a clinician is not a prescribing professional, feedback concerning medication often comes to them. Familiarity with medications fosters client confidence in the clinician. Furthermore, some side effects directly impact the client's progress and response to therapy. Two examples illustrate this point. First, a client having marital problems who develops a lack of sexual desire as a result of Zoloft places additional strain on the relationship; and second a client already dealing with self-esteem problems may become despondent about the added burden of weight gain caused by the drug.

Medication side effects can also make if difficult to interpret client progress. For example, side effects such as emotional flattening and irritability or restlessness resemble psychiatric symptoms of depression or a worsening of anxiety. Is a client who suddenly becomes confused and unable to remember things suffering a dissociative episode or a toxic level of medication? Understanding medication helps the clinician to make accurate interpretations of symptoms.

The clinician should specifically inquire about the client's response to medication and ask about side effects. Such dialogue could result in a recommendation for the client to contact the prescribing professional and also conveys interest in the entirety of client treatment.

Safety

There is no greater concern in the helping relationship than safety of the client. Psychiatric medications are generally safe if taken as prescribed and monitored closely by a medically trained professional. The clinician should emphasize the importance of medical supervision to the client. The most obvious safety issue is suicidal thoughts. The clinician should always inquire about suicidal thoughts and this becomes especially important for the client taking a potentially lethal medication such as tricyclic antidepressants. It is essential to be aware that side effects such as severe anxiety associated with akathisia can result in suicide attempts. Concerns about suicide in a client taking medication need to be dealt with promptly. It is helpful to have established protocols for handling suicidal or other psychiatric emergencies.

Issues of possible misuse and dependence may also be a safety concern. The clinician may become aware of specific vulnerabilities of dependence and abuse. Being excessively medicated because of abuse or excessive drug dosage places the client at risk for accidents and impairs the counseling process.

Abrupt discontinuation of medication can also be a safety risk. Medications should generally be discontinued gradually and under the supervision of the prescribing professional.

Concerns about side effects such as sedation, excessive anxiety, medication misuse, or poor response need to be communicated to the prescribing professional either by the client or with the client's consent. A collaborative approach to the client's care is essential when addressing issues of safety (Coyle, 1999).

Attitudes

Attitudes toward medication are important because many clients have concerns about "being dependent" on medicine or using it as a crutch. Alternatively, some clients become overly dependent on medication and view it as the solution to any obstacle experienced during the counseling process. The clinician may need to explore perceived benefits and risks of medication with clients. The attitude of the clinician may also be an issue. Some clinicians do not believe in medication or do not want to be involved in cases complicated by medication. Others may believe medication is useful, even necessary, but feel the value of counseling competes with medication benefit. However, given the developmental, cultural, and psychosocial context in which mental health problems unfold, pharmacotherapy alone is usually not sufficient. Most research suggests a multimodal approach, stressing the importance of counseling and medication for problems such as anxiety and depression (de Jonghe, Kool, van Aalst, Dekker, & Peen, 2001).

Clients who resist the idea of medication but who clearly have not been able to respond to counseling need to be informed of the limitations and risks of counseling alone. It is difficult to benefit from group therapy or to practice new skills with others when extreme social withdrawal or severe anxiety is a primary symptom of a major mental disorder. Clients previously unable to participate in counseling due to symptom severity may benefit from counseling once treated with appropriate medication.

Clients requiring long-term medication may have concerns about being dependent on medication. The need for long-term maintenance is an issue that arises in the course of working with some clients with a serious mental illness (e.g., schizophrenia, recurrent depression). Sometimes, family members also need support and information to facilitate coping with the client's need for psychiatric medication.

Impact of Psychiatric Medications on the Counseling Process

A client may become sluggish, sedated, or just complain of feeling less alert while on psychiatric medications. In addition, memory can be impaired as a result of medication side effects. This can interfere with the client's capacity to engage in self-reflection and can retard motivation for change. Because much of the counseling process involves accessing memories, rethinking experiences, and processing feelings about one's personal life situation, these side effects can potentially interfere with the counseling process.

There is also the risk that as the medication helps to improve severe symptomatology, the client may lose motivation to continue in the counseling relationship. The opposite is also a possibility: The client may be reluctant to accept the help of medication, but may be too symptomatic to really benefit fully from counseling. A balance is obviously preferred in either scenario.

The issue of diagnostic confusion can also arise during the course of a trial on medication. For instance, a patient with a history of depression becoming manic while taking an antidepressant suggests bipolar disorder. Problems in living can be conceptualized in many ways and confusion can occur for both client and clinician when medication seems to relieve many of the symptoms that initially prompted counseling. Some cases are clear-cut such as the depressed client who responds to medication but has a number of life issues and personality characteristics that perpetuate the depressed mood. For instance, a depressed client who is very passive and dependent and in an unfullfilling relationship clearly needs to work on issues maintaining his or her vulnerability to depression. Other cases are less clear and can be frustrating for the clinician in maintaining clarity about the client's needs.

Referral, Consultation, and Interdisciplinary Collaboration

Clients with severe symptoms that prevent effective psychotherapy; whose symptoms fail to respond to an adequate trial of psychotherapy; and those with chronic or recurrent depression, need to be evaluated for psychiatric medication. Early, aggressive treatment is required because poor outcome, comorbid conditions, and high risk of suicide and substance abuse frequently accompany these recurrent disorders.

Opportunities to work with clients can be enhanced through appropriate consultation and collaboration with other mental health professionals. Interdisciplinary collaboration expands the skills of clinicians and demonstrates the commitment of professional clinicians to being an active presence in promoting the mental health of the public. This section has addressed some of the issues surrounding the use of medication as an adjunct to the counseling process and will hopefully stimulate further thinking about the complex issues of mental health problems with steadily increasing data about biological aspects of mental processes.

COUNSELING POINTS

- Family assessment tools that highlight cultural and health aspects of families lead to more therapeutic alliance, collaboration, and better health outcomes for families.

- Clinicians and families can benefit from discussing the use of medications and understanding their effect on treatment.

- Clinicians who do not dispense medications must be aware of the legal and ethical issues accompanying their use.

7

Family Health Counseling, Counseling in Disasters, Health Interventions, and Reimbursement with Families of Diverse Cultures

Ruth P. Cox, Ken Farr, and Eddie Parrish

FAMILY HEALTH COUNSELING

Family health counseling can be divided into the following four phases: family assessment, treatment plan, family interventions, and evaluation. This is not a linear process but rather a reflexive flow between the stages depending on changes that occur within the family system during treatment. As new information is discovered, re-assessment is done that may necessitate a new treatment plan and interventions.

Development of a Therapeutic Relationship with Multicultural Families

There has been discussion in the literature concerning the *cultural compatibility hypothesis* that suggests that racial/ethnic similarity in turn reinforces the client–family–therapist therapeutic relationship (Paniagua, 1994). However, the overall conclusion suggested by research is that the race or ethnicity of the clinician has no effect on the outcome of treatment (Sue, 1988; Sue, Fujino, Hu, Takeuchi, & Zane, 1991). Futhermore, Sue advised that racial match may lead to a cultural mismatch. On the other hand, Sue suggested that racial mismatches do not necessarily imply cultural mismatches. This is because clinicians and clients from different racial groups may share similar values, lifestyles, and experiences. Conversely, clinicians and clients may share the same racial group, but may not share the same ethnicity—highly acculturated Hispanic clinicians working with less acculturated Hispanic families may result in a cultural mismatch, regardless of the fact that both are of the same racial group. White clinicians working with a highly acculturated Hispanic family may result in a cultural match—both share the same Western culture, values, and traditions. Due to the hostility between some Asian nations (i.e., wars between Chinese and Japanese, Japanese and Koreans), it may not be therapeutic to apply the cultural compatibility hypothesis.

Due to the problems sighted with the cultural compatibility hypothesis, an alternative hypothesis, the *universalistic argument*, has been proposed (Dana, 1993). This hypothesis suggests that effective assessment and treatment are the same across all multicultural groups, independent of the issue of client/family/clinician racial/ethnic differences or similarities.

This hypothesis proposes that what is relevant in the assessment and treatment of multicultural groups is evidence that the therapist can display both cultural sensitivity (i.e., awareness of cultural variables that may affect assessment and treatment) and cultural competence (i.e., translation of this awareness into behavior leading to effective assessment and treatment of the particular multicultural group). (Paniagua, 1994, p. 7)

Thus, White clinicians are as effective as Asian clinicians in the assessment and treatment of Asian clients and families as long as these two qualities are evidenced in clinical practice.

Furthermore, the fact that clinicians and families share the same race and ethnicity does not guarantee the effectiveness of assessment and treatment. Regardless of the shared race/ethnicity, clinicians are still called on to show evidence of sensitivity and competence to enhance assessment and treatment. The universalistic argument also includes the concepts of *credibility* and *giving* (Sue & Sue, 1990). Credibility is the client and family's perception that the clinician is effective and trustworthy. Giving deals with family's recognition that the clinician has provided something of value in the family–clinician relationship. In summary, the ability of the clinician to be culturally competent during assessment and treatment of multicultural families is more important than any similarity in the client's, family's, and clinician's racial or ethnic similarity.

Supervision and Training for Clinical Practice with Multicultural Families

Monitoring of clinical practice is often directly proportional to the efficacy and quality of the treatment outcomes. Due to the vast number of treatment options, adjunctive therapy options, and organizations that provide treatments, ongoing training provides an opportunity for beginning and seasoned clinicians to "hone skills that are necessary to work with individuals, couples, and families" (Helmeke & Prouty, 2001, p. 535). Supervision and training provides an arena to increase clinicians' awareness of and interaction with their own biases and assumptions (gender, sexual identity, cultural/ethnic, family of origin). This is essential as there is an ongoing process of clinicians' own views and assumptions impacting their manners and interactions with families during treatment.

Most states now require evidence of ongoing training and continuing education in order to renew a license. The number of hours and type of continuing education training varies with each state. With some licensing boards, there are often requirements that specify that a certain number of hours must be obtained in certain areas. For example, in one state, the renewal of a marriage and family therapy license requires forty hours, with ten hours specific to the clinical practice of marriage and family therapy, three hours in professional ethics, and if one is an approved supervisor, five hours related to supervision. Some organizations require supervision and training as a requirement for employment that may be either above or below that required for licensure. Clinicians must be aware of the requirements for their particular license and should know that these requirements are different from state to state.

Family Assessment

The assessment process begins with the first contact within the context of the therapist–client–family relationship. Assessment provides the therapist, client, and family an opportunity for a culturally competent dialogue about how they view problems in their system. It is particularly important to view the family and its spirituality embedded in a circular process between the larger culture and the family ethnicy. Through assessment, therapists organize their thinking about the family system. The Family Functioning and Health Assessment (with genogram) and ecomap discussed earlier assist clinicians in understanding the family system within its cultural context.

During the assessment process using the Family Functioning and Health Assessment, the clinician asks questions in each of the assessment categories to initiate an understanding of the client's and family's view of the problem. Using the ecomap assists the therapist and family to expand their view of the family into its environment. How, when, and to whom questions are asked is directed by the cultural/ethnic values of the family. These questions may be asked when the client and family are all together, when several family members come to visit, or may be asked of the client if family members are not available during treatment. Table 3.6 gives examples of questions used when initiating a constructive dialogue. The therapist can alter the questions to include dialoguing with a family member, multiple members, or representatives from various agencies or institutions involved with the family. All of this information provides information for the genogram and ecomap, which is continually updated as new information is discovered.

Legal and Ethical Issues

During the assessment process, clinicians must consider what legal and ethical issues might be involved as the family discourses about problems, such as divorce, child custody, domestic violence, child abuse, and mediation. Many of these issues will depend on the laws of a particular region or state and ethics concerning ethical codes, confidentiality, and privileged communication (Riley, Sargent, Hartwell, & Patterson, 1997). Clinicians can expand their understanding of legal and ethical issues through cooperation with other professionals, such as lawyers, related to public policy. This will help with understanding conceptual/practical differences between professions with the outcome of professionals better able to use each other's expertise more effectively and better able to understand the client and family's experience with the legal system. Moreover, clinicians also must be aware of new situations that advancing technology bring to treatment, which require a different view of ethical, legal, and social implications (AAMFT, 2001).

For example, the Human Genome Project has provided a working draft of the human genome and many genetic technologies have been developed. This brings forth questions such as, if the family suspects a genetic disorder within their family heritage, should predictive testing for genetic disease be done when there is no treatment for the disease? Another issue might deal with mental illness. There is strong support for the heritability of mental illness although multiple genes are probably involved rather than one gene (State, Lombroso, Pauls, & Leckman, 2000). If there is a history of mental illness within the family, questions might revolve around obtaining genetic testing early in life versus examining environmental factors that contribute to the expression of the disorder determined by the genes. These are new areas of discourse on which clinicians must be ready to embark.

Treatment Plan

Healthy Families

Healthy families are unlikely to present themselves for assistance at traditional mental health facilities. Therefore, the clinician likely will meet healthy families in counseling settings such as health promotional and health maintenance programs. Areas for these families would likely focus on enrichment of existing strengths, enhancing parenting skills, disease preventive measures, health promotion, and personal enrichment.

Problem Families

Families who present at mental health centers, community health facilities, or inpatient facilities are more often those with problems. Families with school-age children and children in college also may deal with school counselors. The clinician can help these families with conflict management, communication skills, problem solving, parenting skills, knowledge regarding present difficulties, education regarding normal growth and development, and information about support groups and available resources for the family. Clinicians can assist clients and families in establishing goals to be accomplished during treatment. Referrals for family therapy may be necessary if supportive interventions do not effect resolution of family difficulties.

Troubled Families

Very troubled families are often encountered in family therapy situations in mental health centers, private therapy, or on in-patient psychiatric units. These families' problems often spill out into their environment. Because of this, other agencies may need to be involved or are already involved at the time of initial contact. When establishing goals with these families, clinicians must consider how these agencies will be involved in the treatment process.

Agency contact may focus on economic issues, protection for one or more family members, report of abuse to a state agency, contacts with police, or actions of a court order. Clinicians can assist these families in finding sources of assistance and arranging for these services. These services may include social welfare agencies, churches/synagogues/mosques, emergency food services, voluntary agencies, support groups, hospices, and community health services.

Initiating Family Interventions

The goal of the team–clinician–client–family therapeutic relationship is the participation of all family members, and others as necessary, in conversations that empower family members to construct their own solutions for their family problems. Clinicians must establish an environment for dialogical conversations—conversations where fixed meanings and behaviors are given room, explored, broadened, shifted, within the family's cultural context, and change occurs (Anderson, 1997; H. Anderson & Goolishian, 1988). For example, conversations related to family spirituality may help the family grasp what *spiritual* means for the family and its members and how this can help in the healing process within the family. The following principles will assist in establishing therapeutic conversations:

1. Inquiry is kept within the boundaries of the stated problem.
2. Multiple and contradictory ideas are explored enthusiastically and respectfully with no judgment of "rightness" or "wrongness."
3. All information is taken seriously, no matter how astonishing, trivial, or peculiar it seems, while showing a respect for, not judgment of, what is said.
4. Because language represents life experiences, clinicians converse with the client and family using their metaphorical language within their cultural context.
5. Arriving at conclusions about family system problems too quickly may prevent the creation of new meanings and change.
6. Questions are used to bring forth new ideas that connect with other new ideas to form solutions to problems (Tomm, 1987, 1988).

7. Clinicians facilitate expressions of *multiple* views about the problem, in the interest of maximizing the creation of new meaning.

8. Clinicians provide an atmosphere where gender differences can be explored.

9. Clinicians facilitate an atmosphere where spiritual/religious resources can be explored within the family unit.

10. Clinicians must be prepared to negotiate and change their views as new information is exposed within the family dialogue.

Clinicians can use four types of questions in conversations when families are trying to create solutions for their problems: linear, strategic, circular, and reflexive (Cox & Davis, 1993; Tomm, 1987, 1988; Tomm & Lannamann, 1988). Table 3.6 identifies the four types of questions with intent and examples for each type.

There may be times when family members are not available, due to living at a distance or death, or do not wish to be involved in working with the client. Clinicians can include the absent family member by conversing within a systemic perspective by asking the client, "What do you think your brother would have said about your mother doing this?" (circular question), or "If your mother had done this differently, what do you think would have happened?" (reflexive question). By talking with the client systemically, other views that provide the opportunity for change become possible.

The Politics of Gender in Clinical Practice

Politics are part of ongoing personal and social relationships—likewise, therapeutic relationships cannot escape the influence of gender. However, this influence is often difficult to see. Until recently, it was unfashionable, perhaps even unethical, to openly acknowledge political agendas within clinical practices (Knudson-Martin, 1997). "As agents unavoidably engaged in the political arena of social change we must consider how our theories and strategies support one agenda or social structure or another and we must make conscious decisions about them" (p. 421). How is the nature and scope of gender differences defined? This is one of the most debated and political topics within gender studies. Conclusions regarding clinical responses to the research and discourse on gender differences differ according to which literature and which political agenda one supports. Because gender and family cannot be separated, clinicians who work with families find themselves in the midst of the co-construction of gender. Therefore, how clinicians respond has political consequences for clients, their families, and society at large.

It is most helpful to clients to "avoid unintentionally reinforcing existing gender biases and inequality, and to encourage personal and relationship patterns that equally serve both genders" (Knudson-Martin, 1997, p. 433). In this process, the clinician's role is to assist clients to make invisible processes visible, thus providing an opportunity for women and men to make conscious decisions regarding their patterned ways of relating. Clinicians can provide this environment by attending to the following:

- Develop sensitivity to how gender affects one's view of experience and relationship structure.
- Do not make the assumption of equality in relationships or assume that there is no gender bias present.
- Being neutral may require an active response in asking each person to accommodate in some way.
- Ask "gendercentic" questions—make gender the topic for circular questions.
- Focus on process—make gender open for invisible patterns being made visible.
- Articulate the issues—help identify and put into words gender construction issues that are presently a problem.
- Externalize—discussing gender can link the problem to the larger culture of collective struggles within a social context and make change more possible.

Dienhart and Avis' (1994) study provides a beginning formulation for a gender-sensitive approach when working with men in treatment. Thirty-six family therapists endorsed 131 interventions as appropriate and effective ways of working with men. Interventions were highly endorsed in the following six categories:

1.0 Developing therapist's perceptual and conceptual skills

2.0 Promoting mutual responsibility

   2.1 Assessment

   2.2 Unbalancing/rebalancing

   2.3 Empowering

   2.4 Reframing

   2.5 Communication skills

3.0 Challenging sterotypical behavior and attitudes

   3.1 Psychoeducation

   3.2 Cognitive restructuring

   3.3 Role reversals

   3.4 Examining family-of-origin issues

   3.5 Direct challenge

4.0 Challenging family's power balance

5.0 Encouraging effective expression in men

6.0 Structuring treatment

   6.1 Scheduling

   6.2 Use of varying treatment modalities

The overall results of the research support a "'connect and challenge' approach, beginning by joining with a man's pain and then challenging his learned patterns of control and power" (p. 413). The panel suggested these approaches rather than the more direct educational or confrontational approaches typical of a traditional masculine model.

Skills for Transcultural/Multicultural Family Counseling

Since the 1970s, mental health counseling, therapy, and family health professionals have increasingly emphasized the need for clinicians to develop mulitcultural–transcultural counseling–therapy competencies (Hanson, 2001; Pedersen, 1991a, 1991b; Sue, Arredondo, & McDavis, 1992; Wright & Leahey, 2000). In the counseling profession, multiculturalism has been deemed a new paradigm, the *fourth force in counseling* (Pedersen, 1991a). Multiculturalism must include differences based on religion, sexual orientation, socioeconomic factors, age, gender, physical (dis)abilities, and levels of acculturation and assimilation (Sue, Ivey, & Pedersen, 1996). This new force of multiculturalism is truly *postmodern* in that it entertains the existence of multiple belief systems and multiple perspectives rather than being based on modernism, an epistemology characterized by rational, linear, positivist, and empirical traditions in Western science (Gonzalez, 1997).

Thus, multiculturalism may encompass *social constructionism* in which meanings and the view of reality are developed through social interaction (networks of social agreements) and *constructivism*, which deals with the construction of personal realities. Based on this postmodern philosophy, several assumptions inherent in multiculturalism when used as a force in counseling and therapy can be identified (Gonzalez, 1997; Sue et al., 1996):

1. Multiculturalism accepts the existence of multiple worldviews. There are multiple alternative means to ask and answer questions about the family besides the logical–positivist paradigm.

2. Multiculturalism embodies social constructionism. Families construct their worlds through social processes, historical, cultural, and social, that use cultural symbols and metaphors.

3. Multiculturalism is contextual. Behavior can only be understood within the context of its occurrence.

4. Multiculturalism offers a "both/and" rather than an "either/or" view of the family's world. This allows for all types of counseling and therapy to exist under the same umbrella, allowing for different views of the same phenomenon.

5. Multiculturalism extols a relational view of language, rather than a representational view. This relational view allows for realities and truths beyond the Western scientific-"modern" tradition.

With this postmodern view and assumptions of multiculturalism, mulitcultural counseling and therapy can be defined (Sue et al., 1998). This is an approach that:

1. Recognizes that all models and theories of assistance originate from a particular cultural context.
2. Refers specifically to a helping relationship in which two or more of the participants are of different cultural backgrounds.
3. Includes any counseling combination that fulfills the definition of culture.
4. Recognizes the use of both Western and non-Western approaches.
5. Is characterized by the clinician's culturally appropriate awareness, knowledge, and skills.

This is a very inclusive definition and may mean different things to different people. Thus, it forces clinicians, who practice from this philosophy, to be clear about their approach with themselves, clients and families, colleagues, and other professionals.

Therefore, to work constructively with clients and their families from a multicultural–transcultural paradigm, the clinician must possess the following skills: *self-knowledge skills,* including personal coping skills, biases and prejudices, resistance to system seductions, and availability for clinical supervision; *assessment skills; therapeutic communication skills,* including knowledge of systems and family theory, family interviewing skills, and teaching/learning principles; *spiritual skills for caregivers; case management skills; collaboration and consultation skills;* and *skills regarding referrals, family support, and resources* (Cox, 1999). These skills are embedded within and influenced by the cultural/ethnic context of the clinician and family.

Self-Knowledge Skills

Clinicians must be able to identify and own their thoughts, beliefs, feelings, actions, and biases that are influenced by their culture and ethnicity before they can understand these in others, especially if the family is culturally different. Clinicians working with families must become aware of their own family dynamics to preclude confusing their own family-of-origin issues with those of their clients and families. Working with families in mental health can be very intense. Therefore, clinicians must attend to health issues through development of personal coping skills such as exercise, nurturance, and support from colleagues and friends.

By using a family-oriented theory, clinicians must learn to think "circularly" rather than linearly (as in cause and effect). Clinicians must constantly resist the idea to view one family member as "the problem" rather than systemically viewing interactions between all family members as sources for family problem solving. The seduction of a unipolar view of seeing one person's view as more "right" than another, must be replaced with multipartiality—the view that all members ideas are equally valuable and justifiable. Clinicians must resist being seduced into adopting sterotypical gender behaviors and attitudes. In many cultural groups, extended family is an important part of the family system— clinicians should let the family define this rather than imposing their own view (Paniagua, 1994). Clinical supervision can assist clinicians in becoming aware of any seductions and increase the effectiveness of their interventions.

Clinicians should not confuse multiculturalism with diversity, as they are not synonymous, although diversity may be a necessary, but not sufficient, condition to achieve the former. *Diversity* is a term used to describe the changing worker characteristics, such as race, ethnicity, gender, sexual orientation, age, religion, and physical ability or disability (Sue et al., 1998). Diversity relates to the presence or absence of numerical symmetry of these differences in our society. Some have advocated a separation between mulitcultural distinctions—reserved only for race, ethnicity, and culture; and diversity—reserved for all other people differences (Arredondo et al., 1996). Clinicians must be mindful of all these variables when understanding families within their full cultural/ethnic context.

Assessment Skills

It is important for the clinician to constantly resist the view of one family member as being "the problem." Instead, the clinician must view systematically the interactions *between* all family members as sources for family problem solving. The family is viewed as a collaborative partner with the clinician in health care problem solving and decision making. Also, clinicians must resist gender and cultural/ethnic sterotyping within the family unit (Pope-Davis & Coleman, 1997). As the clinician uses a family assessment guide effectively and efficiently, the most complete information can be available to both the clinician and family as decisions are made based on the family's self-discovery of strengths and resources. Due to cultural differences (particularly Hispanics), this information may need to be collected over time rather than collecting a large amount during the first meeting (Paniagua, 1994). Clinicians and family members become aware of community institutions and agencies that are involved with the family. Translators are an option with families who have limited English proficiency (Paniagua, 1994; guidelines for the use of translators can be found on pp. 12–13). The possibility of overdiagnosing clients from any of the multicultural groups is an issue clinicians should always keep in mind. In this manner, all aspects of information gathering are "'family perceived' as well as 'professional perceived'. The intent of the partnership here is to clarify discrepant views and to discover fresh alternatives for action" (Lapp, Diemert, Enestvedt, 1993, p. 311).

Therapeutic Communication Skills

Clinicians, having a working knowledge of systems, culture, ethnicity, spirituality, and family theories concepts, are provided then with a conceptional framework as a basis for culturally competent interventions. This knowledge includes the belief that families are functioning the best that they can, families can solve their own problems, strengths exist in all families, parents are doing the best job they can, no one is to blame for the family problems, and people act in unconstructive ways when protecting and shielding themselves from painful interactions.

Family interviewing skills include the ability to interact simultaneously with all family members with the same amount of respect and nonjudgment, being aware of gender and culture sterotyping, while working on the stated problem (e.g., when one family member has been identified as the perpetrator of violent acts). Clinicians' attention must be given to observing the interactions between and among members of the system, and at times between agencies and institutions outside the family, rather than focusing on the actions of one individual. Additionally, clinicians must conceptualize their observations of the family as a system existing within a culture and legal system rather than individuals interacting with one another. Interventions are based on the information received from the client and family within their cultural context and from institutions outside the family unit when appropriate. New information forms the basis for future observations and hypotheses about the family. The interviewing process is a circular phenomenon between the clinician, client, family, and their environment (Wright & Leahey, 1994). Clinicians need knowledge of various teaching strategies and learning principles because families do not learn information in the same way and learning may be culturally and gender specific.

Spiritual Skills for Caregivers

Families have identified that facilitative attitudes are one method of coping with a family member with a problem (Doornbos, 1997). Facilitative attitudes include tolerance, patience, acceptance, nonreactiveness, forgiveness, love, encouragement, and hopefulness. These attitudes flow out of the spiritual dimension of individuals (Carson, 1989). The clinician can intervene effectively with family caregivers by providing spiritual care. Skills include entering into a relationship with the caregiver, becoming a companion in his or her journey, and sharing the caregiver's emotions such as pain, anger, or sadness (Carson, 1989).

Case Management Skills

Clinicians work with family systems holistically by viewing aspects within as well as outside the family in larger systems, such as the community, schools, churches/synagogues/mosques, and governments. This allows clinicians to assist families in dealing with the many problems they face and provide crisis intervention when necessary. Therefore, clinicians working with families are in an excellent position to serve as case managers.

Collaboration and Consultation Skills

Clinicians must work effectively as peers with colleagues in providing care for families and meeting family goals. Through collaboration, clinicians work with other disciplines toward family outcomes. Clinicians who are knowledgeable about families can consult with other health professionals, school boards, advisory boards, and work with legislators concerning family issues.

Collaboration skills have been identified by McDaniel and Campbell (1996). The following is a list of those that clinicians need when working with families and other agencies:

1. Maintain attention to collaborative values
   - Focus primarily on capacities as opposed to deficits
   - Promote universal access to health care
   - Empower, educate, and learn from families
   - Value interdependency
2. Become accountable for the use of resources
   - Track statistics and outcomes
3. Discuss, monitor, and deal with issues of shared power among professionals, and between professionals, clients, and families
   - Create space for everyone to have a place in the discourse
   - Examine the relationship between power and helping professions, between competition and collaboration
   - Develop case-specific leadership, dependent on the needs of the client and the context of the case
   - Learn to be both a leader and a follower
   - Develop the ability to talk about differences
4. Examine issues of culture, race, class, and disabilities in health care
   - Make services culturally responsive
   - Develop ways to accept and support differences
   - Examine cultural countertransference
5. Learn to enhance others' competencies
6. Attend to issues of spirituality

Skills for Referrals, Family Support, and Resources

Referrals are often necessary when working with troubled families as many of their needs and tasks are not being met. Clinicians must have knowledge of and necessary skill to support families as they enter the desired system for assistance.

Evaluation

Outcomes of working with clients and their families can be measured by (a) comparing present family functioning with the assessment criteria in the Family Health and Functioning Assessment model when the family started in treatment, (b) determining whether treatment goals have been met, and (c) concluding whether clients and families have created new meanings and solutions for present problems. Periodically throughout the treatment process, the clinician and family system together must evaluate their progress toward the resolution of their present problems. Where appropriate, clinicians can assist clients and families in the reformulation of goals and the creation of post-treatment goals that will be worked toward after discharge from an inpatient unit. Clinicians may make themselves available for consultation with families after discharge to support the continuation of changes that have been initiated during hospitalization. Clinicians can serve as a resource for referral to service agencies and organizations that will assist families post-discharge.

RESEARCH FOCUS—A NEED FOR EVIDENCE-BASED TREATMENTS

Historically, much of the research done in the mental health field has had little applicability in the real world of treatment. More recently, there has been a shift to test not only the efficacy of clinical interventions, but to assess the applicability of these interventions in real-world situations ("Empirically Validated," 2000). Institutions like the National Institute of Mental Health (NIMH) and the National Institute on Drug Abuse (NIDA) have been supporting *effectiveness* and *translational research*.

Effectiveness research focuses on using the findings from clinical trails (i.e., efficacy research) to see how these work in clinical practice. As this type of research limits the variables that may interfere with the intervention being tested, it is problematic for the real world as these very variables are often the reasons that clients seek treatment. Therefore, the consequence of this type of research is that the interventions proved to work in clinical trials "have limited utility outside the laboratory or study site" ("Empirically Validated," 2000, p. 22).

In recognizing this as a problem, the NIMH has begun to focus not only on the application of efficacious treatments in clinical practice, but also on translational research, sometimes called transportational research. This type of research is focused on identifying the best ways to get clinicians to use treatments shown effective with particular populations. "We know very little about the obstacles and impediments to successful implementation of effective treatments and even less about the fidelity to these interventions in 'real world' settings" (p. 22).

In the near future, it will be unacceptable to utilize treatment approaches that have not been empirically validated. Clinicians may find that they will not be reimbursed by insurance if the treatment plan does not use validated treatment methods. The area of child and adolescent family therapy has several approaches that have empirical support. These include (with original developers in parentheses): Multisystem Therapy (Bourduin & Henggler); Multidimensional Family Therapy (Liddle); Functional Family Therapy (Alexander); Brief Strategic Family Therapy (Szapocznik) ("Empirically Validated," 2000); and the Center for Substance Abuse Prevention's Prevention Enhancement Protocols System (Kumpfer & Kaftarian) (Kumpfer & Kaftarian, 2000).

The majority of effective treatments are individually focused interventions, such as Anger Coping Management, Problem Solving Skill Training and Rational Emotive Therapy. Others have been parent focused interventions, including Videotape Modeling, Parent–Child Interaction Therapy, and Parent Training Program. Several community-based interventions have been useful, such as intensive case management, home-based treatments, therapeutic foster care, and group homes. As more treatment models are found to be effective, the next steps would be to discern what treatments are best of what types of problems and with what populations.

REIMBURSEMENT FOR SERVICES

Third-party payment for mental health services is generally based on the medical model of understanding and documenting client problems and the treatment of those problems. Graduate education varies greatly in the numerous programs that train clinicians. The various programs emphasize different aspects of treatment ranging from focusing on personal growth to treating severe psychopathology. Clinicians whose educational training emphasized personal growth may be less comfortable with the medical model based on criteria found in the *Diagnostic and Statistical Manual of Mental Disorders, Fourth Edition, Text Revision (DSM-IV-TR;* APA, 2000a) than those whose education encompasses more chronic mental health concerns and specific Axis I and Axis II issues. Clinicians whose education does not include a pathology model may conduct and document treatment in a manner that is therapeutically beneficial, but may not be reimbursable by current third-party standards. Documentation training will help ease this discrepancy.

Reimbursement for therapy depends on (a) educational discipline and level of preparation; (b) state and federal laws, rules, and regulations; and (c) state and federal licensure and certification laws, rules, and regulations. Each state varies greatly. When conflict arises between state and federal regulations, federal regulations supercede state regulations only when the third-party reimbursing agency is a federal program. State laws regulating and delineating scope of practice supercede federal regulations within each state.

Clear and thorough documentation enables clinicians from all schools of thought and third-party payors to track therapeutic progress. Relatively few insurance companies clearly depict their criteria for reimbursement for mental health services. The medical model requires "medical necessity" to qualify for third-party payment. Third-party payors have varying requirements for reimbursement of services, depending on the state in which the service is provided and the company that is the third-party payor. General guidelines include the following:

1. Services should be medically or therapeutically necessary.
2. Services should be directed at a diagnosable mental illness or disorder (*DSM-IV-TR* coded disorder).
3. Services should be consistent with the diagnosis and degree of impairment.
4. There should be documentation of reasonable progress consistent with the treatment of the disorder.
5. A treatment plan must be developed, including specific discharge criteria written in behavioral terms.
6. Services must be specifically directed toward the *DSM-IV-TR* diagnosis.
7. If services are to be continued, there should be documented evidence of continued impairment.
8. Progress notes should reflect the treatment plan's stated goals and objectives.

Clinicians should insist that any copayments the client is required to pay are collected or arrangements for the payment of copayments should be made. When delivering therapy services to clients of diverse cultural and socioeconomic backgrounds, it may be necessary to reinforce that therapy is a service that is to reimbursed in the society and culture of the United States. Not to insist on reimbursement and payment of required copayments devalues therapy and encourages helplessness, dependency, and a lack of responsibility to deal with personal problems.

Reimbursement requires detailed investigation by each clinician into the state and federal laws that regulate a particular clinician's practice. A thorough written client assessment, exact diagnosis, complete treatment plan, and progress notes addressing each session, including goal, intervention, outcome, and plan should be completed and available for third-party payor review.

FAMILY COUNSELING IN DISASTERS

Over the past few years, the realities of disasters in the United States and the world have been brought to the forefront and the public's attention by the news media. Global access to the Internet has made it possible to know, at any time, the up-to-the-minute status of any event in the world. On September 11, 2001, in the United States, the public and world viewed as the World Trade Center's towers were attacked by two hijacked public aircraft. The public, present and by media, viewed as both World Trade Center towers cascaded onto themselves into the depths of New York City. Two thousand eight hundred twenty-three persons, including firemen and police, lost their lives in this disaster (After 260 Grim Days, 2002). One thousand seven hundred twenty-one of those lost have yet to be found. Moreover, their bodies will never be recovered from the mountain of debris, as 1.8 million tons of debris have been removed and the ground zero recovery effort ended on May 30, 2002.

A disaster is defined as an event that involves destruction of property, includes injury and/or loss of life, and affects a large population and is shared by many families. (U.S. Department of Health & Human Services, 1995, p. 1). Disasters are sudden events that occur out of the realm of normal human experience. From a psychological view, disasters are traumatic enough to induce stress in any person, regardless of previous experience or function with a diversity of disasters. Disasters are usually classified as natural or human-caused. Natural disasters are caused by a force of nature (i.e., earthquakes, hurricanes, fires, floods), with no one to blame, in various locations with a high amount of postdisaster distress (U.S. Department of Health & Human Services, 1995). On the other hand, human-caused disasters are caused by human error and/ or malfunctioning technology (i.e., airplane crashes, major chemical spills, nuclear reactor accidents, bombings, terrorism, civil unrest), with specific persons, governments, or businesses to blame, with little or no advanced warning in locations that may be inaccessible to rescuers and unfamiliar to survivors, and have a higher level of postdisaster stress than natural disasters. This higher level of stress is often felt by family members not involved in the disaster. Some disasters can be due to a combination of causes, such as an airplane crash due to poor weather conditions.

The aftermath of a disaster is serious and has widespread physical and emotional sequella. Furthermore, "the emotional impact of a disaster often persists well after the physical impact" (U.S. Department of Health & Human Services, 1995, p. vii). Children are particularly hardhit by disasters. Effects of the disaster may evidence themselves at home, school, and/or in the community. These are usually normal reactions to an abnormal event. If assistance is not given to children and their families, the effects of the disaster can turn into problems for children, such as school truancy and behavior problems, and in the community, such as illegal acts, disobeying curfews, and delinquency. Adults and children can suffer symptoms of dissociation (Steinberg, 2000/ 2001) and post-traumatic stress, which when it affects their ability to function, can be termed *post-traumatic stress disorder* (PTSD); (APA, 2000a).

Effects on a Community

As families do not live in a vacuum. It is important to consider the effects of a disaster within the context of the community in which the family and its extended members reside (U.S. Department of Health & Human Services, 1995). Disasters will differ in their effects based on scope, intensity, and the characteristics of the predisaster community, family, and individual personalities. The effects of the disaster are often widespread and include the following:

destruction of infrastructure

absence of electricity, sanitation, and potable water

destruction of contact with the outside world through roadways, bridges, and phones

dissipation of community cohesion due to death and injury

vulnerability and exploitation due to disaster and media sensationalism

potential for reoccurrence

Cultural, Ethnic, and Spiritual Considerations for Families in Disasters

Although little research has been done to determine the unique impact of disasters on children and families of a specific culture/ethnic group, there is some information available showing differences (Joyner & Swenson, 1993; Sugar, 1992a). In all phases of a disaster, leaders of different cultural/ethnic groups must be available to provide family contact within the community. Information needed by the different groups must be provided in a language appropriate to all groups of families within the community.

As spirituality may be a resource for families when coping with, and recovering from a disaster and its aftermath, clergy of all denominations, churches, synagogues, and mosques must become active with families in the community during and after a disaster. Collaboration between health care professionals and the clergy of all denominations should be established to assist families in coping with a disaster.

General Effects on Families and Children/Adolescents

Clinicians must remember that in a disaster, in most cases, families and children are having normal reactions to an abnormal event. It is often easier for parents to seek treatment for their children than to seek treatment for themselves. Moreover, parents may present a symptomatic child as an entry into the health care system when seeking care for themselves. Clinicians can assure parents that the children will be cared for and then engage parents in dialogue about their health care needs. This is essential so that parents are then available to care for their children—analogous to parents putting on an oxygen mask in an airplane and then putting on the child's mask.

Adequate parental coping in a disaster is a factor in children's coping. Parental response to a disaster correlates well with that of the child (U.S. Department of Health & Human Services, 1995). Therefore, it is most helpful if parents deal with the disaster in as healthy a way as possible. However, preexisting family conflicts or pathology may impede adaptation to life changes after a disaster. Family recovery may be impeded by an increase in domestic violence, parental alcoholism, and/or substance abuse. If a parent is overprotective or relies too heavily on the child for support, a child's personal resolution of the effects of the disaster may be delayed.

Generally, children's reaction to a disaster is dependent on the following factors (U.S. Department of Health & Human Services, 1995, pp. 12–13):

- proximity to the impact zone
- awareness of the disaster
- physical injury sustained
- amount of disability
- witnessing of injury or death of family members or friends
- perceived or actual life threat
- duration of life disruption
- familiar and personal property loss
- parental reactions and extent of familial disruptions
- child's predisaster state
- probability of recurrence

Moreover, the following five responses are seen in children who have dealt with loss, been exposed to trauma, and had a disruption of their routine:

1. increased dependency
2. nightmares
3. regression in developmental achievements
4. specific fears about reminders of the disaster (i.e., a toy airplane if the child was in a plane crash)
5. demonstration of the disaster via posttraumatic play and reenachments

These responses usually last for a month or so after the disaster and vary with age and gender (Sugar, 1992b). Girls may appear more distressed, are more verbal about their emotions, ask more questions, and think about the disaster more often than boys. Boys take longer than girls to recover and may display more aggressive, antisocial, and violent behaviors. All members of the family are at risk for feelings of anxiety and depression after a disaster. If these persist, referral to counseling may be appropriate for the whole family and parents can consult with their primary care physician concerning their reactions to the disaster.

Pre-existing Health Risk Factors Affecting Health Care During and After a Disaster

In order to provide the most comprehensive care, clinicians must know as much as possible about the health of all family members. For example, there may be pre-existing physical disabilities or psychopathology with children or other family members. In dysfunctional families, alcohol and/or substance abuse may be the norm. Adults and children with developmental disorders may need additional care due to disruption of care or worsening of their condition/s during and after a disaster. These children and families should be of high priority when care is provided. Those with exacerbation of pre-existing mental and/or physical problems should be referred back to their previous clinician for specific treatment within their community setting.

Families in which a child is born immediately before or during the disaster, or who are in the early stages of nursing, bonding, and attachment, may need special attention. New mothers may need assistance with accessing and acquiring proper food, water, formula, and supplies due to the added stressors of the disaster.

Disruption on Normal Patterns of Life After a Disaster

One of the most prominent features of a disaster is its disruption of the lives of children and their families, whether through injury, death, or destruction of the home, school, or community. Children of all ages are affected by the loss of reliability, cohesion, and predictability in their lives (Sugar, 1992a). Toddlers respond with increased dependency, whereas school-age children show evidence of the disaster with talk and play about the trauma, hostility to peers and family, and avoidance of previously enjoyable activities. Adolescents may withdraw, may have decreased interests, or may experience fatigue, hypertension, and hostility. Many children experience sleep disturbance (i.e., insomnia), resistance to bedtime, refusal to sleep alone, early rising or excessive sleep. With teenagers, increased substance abuse, amenorrhea, and pregnancy can occur.

In dealing with these disruptions in the normal patterns of live, clinicians can direct parents to provide as much routine, predictable scheduling as possible for the family. For instance, with sleep disturbance, flexibility is needed simultaneously with a routine bed schedule. Discipline should be re-established to what was usual before the disaster. Children who have daytime distress may need to be referred to their primary care physician in consultation with a mental health practitioner—this will also apply to adult members of the family.

Behavioral Reactions to a Disaster

Toddlers and preschoolers may show hostile behaviors such as hitting, biting, or pinching, whereas school-age children may fight with their peers. Adolescents may become delinquent or excessively rebellious, often acting out these behaviors within the community setting. Interventions with younger children may incorporate limit setting to bring about the desired change in behavior. With adolescents, involvement in rebuilding the community, helping the elderly, or working with younger children may assist them in dealing with their feelings from the disaster. Preteens and adolescents may find groups, such as Scouts or school clubs, for guided, informal discussions of their thoughts and feelings.

Repetitious behaviors may be seen in the play of toddlers and preschoolers after a disaster. Children will re-enact the disaster as a coping mechanism, but with a different outcome or the child or family member may be a hero. Other, more intrusive repetitious behaviors may occur, such as recurrent nightmares, trauma-specific flashbacks, and distress with reminders of the disaster event. Such intrusions can affect concentration and may be frightening. Posttrauma play and re-enactments show that the child is still involved with the disaster, yet on the other hand, this play assists in dispelling the traumatic effects of the disaster and is therefore therapeutic for the child.

Regressive behaviors, such as separation anxiety, enuresis, encorpresis, thumb-sucking, loss of acquired speech, increased clinging and whining, fear of the darkness, competition for attention, and extreme dependency, are common during and after a disaster. These regressive symptoms are usually short-lived immediately following the disaster. Therefore, parents should be advised that no punishment or shame should be attached to these behaviors during this time. If the symptoms last more than a few weeks, consultation with the family primary care physician and counseling for the child and family should be sought. However, return to a routine and stable household and the passage of time usually rectify these behaviors.

Post-Traumatic Stress Disorder

PTSD can be seen in children and adults following any type of trauma, such as a disaster. However, not all children show all the symptoms and thus do not develop the full disorder. Some children may have a delayed reaction to the disaster, seeming to do well in the midst of the event and shortly thereafter. If the symptoms persist for at least two days but no longer than four weeks, the person may have an acute stress disorder (APA, 2000a). However, if the symptoms are related to re-experiencing the event and persist for four weeks, then the child or adult may be experiencing PTSD. Counseling should be sought and collaboration with the primary care physician is also recommended.

POSSIBLE RESOURCES DURING A DISASTER

Many resources are available during a disaster. All state and local governments have disaster plans that are appropriate for those types of disasters most likely to strike in the area. The American Red Cross is available to help with all disasters that occur within the geographic boundaries of the continental United States and its territories.

At the local and state level the following resources are available:

- Mental health services for children and their families.
- School guidance programs and out-of-home child-care centers.
- American Red Cross provides immediate basic need (food, clothing, shelter).
- Professional organizations provide services and may be networking with the American Red Cross (i.e, American Association for Marriage and Family Therapy, American Psychological Association).
- Religious organizations (i.e., churches, synagogues, and mosques have types of disaster relief programs).
- Universities and medical schools may provide practitioners—caution must be taken that these are responders who can deal with trauma.
- Media, such as television, radio, and newspapers, provide listings of available resources and supports (U.S. Department of Health & Human Services, 1995).

At the national level, the following resources are available:

- Federal Emergency Management Agency (FEMA), which provides logistical and financial assistance to individuals, businesses, and communities after an officially declared disaster.
- Center for Mental Health Services-Emergency Services and Disaster Relief Branch provides crisis counseling to disaster survivors and provides consultation regarding disaster preparedness.
- Centers for Disease Control and Prevention provides epidemiologic intelligence, health surveys, and broad-based consultation.
- Professional organizations have produced handouts useful in disasters, produced research, and developed networks of qualified consultants (i.e., American Association for Marriage and Family Therapy, American Psychological Association, American Academy of Child and Adolescent Psychiatry, National Academy of School Psychologists, American Nurses Association, American Academy of Pediatrics) (U.S. Department of Health & Human Services, 1995).

FAMILY AND COMMUNITY INTERVENTIONS AFTER DISASTERS

Primary Care Physicians

Primary care physicians can be one of the major sources of information, support, and interventions for children, families, and communities after a disaster (U.S. Department of Health & Human Services, 1995). Their role includes, but is not limited to, the following:

- Availability to parents.
- Instructing parents about behaviors to look for in children after a disaster.
- Providing referrals for families requiring mental health or other services.

- Consultating with schools.
- Identifying psychiatric or physical signs of stress in all children and their families.

During this time, physicians should also be aware of their personal reaction to the disaster. They may be dealing with their own personal losses and problems. Their office or residence may have been damaged or destroyed during the disaster. They may have been providing services throughout the time of the disaster. They may have had clients die during the disaster and may be mentally and physically exhausted. Help in coping with the aftermath of the disaster may include speaking with colleagues, support groups, and spiritual counseling.

Schools

It is extremely important that primary care physicians or other health care workers who are working with the family collaborate with the school. After a disaster, schools are a natural site for monitoring children's behaviors as they deal with the aftermath of the disaster, either when schools are used as temporary shelters or are functional again. Schools are a place where the following can occur:

- Education of school staff about normal behavior to expect in their students.
- Screening for high-risk problems.
- Assembling a list of referral sources.
- Counseling programs for families.
- Disseminating written information for parents and students.
- Consulting services to deal with death and grieving for students and school staff.

Media

Primary care physicians and mental health professionals can produce public service announcements to assist families with care and services after a disaster. Health clinicians can provide guidance through discussing psychosocial and physical sequelae of disasters for children and their families through the radio and television and by setting up hotlines. Clinicians can advocate for families by discouraging inappropriate or distressing media attention dealing with the disaster.

Religious Organizations

Primary care physicians and mental health professionals can collaborate with clergy of all faiths to assist individuals and families in coping with death, disaster, grief, mourning, and loss. Health professionals can speak with different faith groups in order to assist them in their specific needs in dealing with outcomes of the disaster.

COUNSELING POINTS

- Cultural sensitivity and competence allow clinicians to work with families irrespective of cultural or ethnic difference between clinicians and families.
- Family health counseling, with all its phases, is a reflexive and recursive process; it is not static.
- Legal and ethical issues affecting treatment must be discussed openly with families.
- Clinicians must be aware of gender issues affecting treatment.
- Clinicians must assess their comfort with the specific skills necessary for transcultural–multicultural counseling.
- Empirically validated treatments are needed for effective treatment.
- Clinicians must be aware of reimbursement issues when working with families.
- Families and communities engaged with disasters must be aware of the multifaceted effects during and after the disaster on families and communities.

8

Transcultural Family Counseling
A Case Study

Ruth P. Cox

FAMILY COUNSELING AND HEALTH INTERVENTIONS WITH THE BELCHER FAMILY

The Belcher family is of Jewish-Catholic Russian-European descent. They were seen in therapy regarding issues related to the oldest daughter in the family. The complete therapy process with the family cannot be reported here. However, examples are given to highlight how the ideas and concepts presented earlier in the book were used in working with this family.

Initial Interviews and Assessment

The Belcher family was seen at the request of the father, Errol, who expressed concern about his oldest daughter who has been married twice. His concern was specific to the spiritual nature in which the grandchildren are being raised. He and his wife wanted to come first, followed by the whole family. The parents were first seen for two sessions (a Bowenian approach) and then the adult children were included. Over several initial interviews, the Family Health and Functioning Assessment, including structure, process, spirituality, and internal and external factors, was completed along with a three-generation genogram (see Figure 3.3; this has had data continuously added as information unfolded) and ecomap (Figure 6.1). Family members completed Olson's FACES-III (see Figure 3.4). Also, Aviva provided information from her previous therapy when married to Mark. Figure 8.1 shows Aviva's family type, using FACES-III, over the years of Aviva's marriages.

Errol and Judy met with the therapist for several sessions regarding their presenting concern over their daughter, Aviva, not bringing up her children in the church. They described a very difficult second divorce from Mark, in which the court had been involved over custody of the children due to possible incest

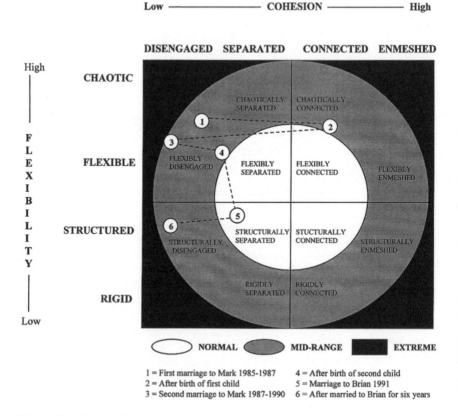

Figure 8.1.   Aviva's Marriages

by Mark, which was never proven. They described heated conflict when Aviva married Mark for the second time. Aviva describes her relationship with Mark as very conflictual. Although Aviva has been married to Brian for several years now, there has been no successful resolution or healing over past, intensely painful events within the family.

Errol and Judy describe the years when the girls (Aviva and Helen) were younger as very pleasant. Although they are both busy professionals, they said they tried to organize their family life so that there was time for themselves with the children. Errol's mother lived with them on occasion after her divorce. Although Errol reports quite a bit of conflict between him and his parents, the girls described a warm relationship with their grandmother. When Aviva became a teenager, she began to be a bit of a "rebel," but they were not too bothered by that. "We figured she would outgrow it." Helen always tried to be helpful in these situations with Aviva, as she never got into trouble. The parents described times when there seemed to be certain "camps" in the household. This caused anger and resentment among different family members. Presently, Helen is a college student and has a boyfriend whom the parents like.

Following is the initial Family Health and Functioning Assessment for the Belcher family including genogram (Figure 3.3), Ecomap (Figure 6.1), and Olson's Circumplex Model with the Belcher Family (Figure 3.4) and with Aviva's marriages (Figure 8.1).

Family Health and Functioning Assessment

I. Family Interview

  A. Demographic and family composition: See genogram, Figure 3.3 (for clarity, not all relationships are shown) and ecomap, Figure 6.1.

  B. Family Interactions

    1. Family Structure

      a. Subsystems: *spousal* and *parental* unit—Errol and Judy; *sibling*—Aviva and Helen; *intergenerational*—paternal grandmother (lived with the family occasionally) and maternal grandmother; and the *social network*—church, hospital, neighborhood, school, and relatives.

      b. Boundaries: *Internal boundaries* are largely open and flexible. Discipline is a matter of lengthy lecture that may or may not result in behavioral change. Different family members tried out the power role but, in the end, Mom or Dad have the power. The family cooperated in many tasks where closeness and affection were encouraged. All report "I love you" was always said. Mom and Dad seem to support each other's as well as their children's goals. During Aviva's stormy teenage years, Helen thinks that the openness and flexibility always practiced backfired, as Aviva rebelled against any discipline or display of authority.

      External boundaries are mostly closed and less flexible. Due to the public nature of Errol's profession, when they are at home away from the public, privacy and locked doors are practiced. Due to busy lives, events are always scheduled and the parents focus on necessary tasks.

      c. Roles: *Father's roles*: analyst, breadwinner, caretaker, decision maker, educator, disciplinarian, friend, and supporter. *Mother's roles*: advocate, breadwinner, caretaker, educator, friend, martyr, nurturer, and supporter. *Aviva's roles*: "black sheep," friend, heavy, scapegoat, and victim. *Helen's roles*: angel, analyst, clown, friend, good child, mediator, mentor, peacekeeper, supporter, and therapist.

      d. Rules: *Procedural rules*: Family eating dinner together when possible (when the children were younger, they always ate together), spending all the holidays together, and keeping others informed of their whereabouts.

      Relational rules: treat each other equally and with respect; be affectionate with each other. Sexuality was discussed openly and questions were always answered.

      e. Triangles: There were two central *triangles*—1: parents and Aviva, 2: Judy, Lilyan (Judy's mother), and Helen (this was and continues to be a warm, positive triad)

   2. Family Process

      a. *Separateness/connectedness*: The family reports an emotional closeness, even when going through some terrible times. There is also a certain level of separateness; Aviva being more separated from the family, especially in her early years. Errol and Judy report that they were closer when the children were younger.

      b. *Enmeshed/disengaged*: The family describes itself as "sticking closely together" (*enmeshed*). They were all connected together, which made seeking independence a difficult task. Aviva said she had to "break out" and break all the rules in an effort to gain her independence and she continues to have difficulty with her father trying to tell her how to deal with her children.

      c. *Communication*: In difficult times, they often communicate to each other through other family members putting an emotional hardship on individuals in the middle. For example, Lilyan would often talk to Judy on Helen's behalf.

      d. *Power*: The parents report an even distribution of power between them, although Aviva gains power through manipulation. Helen, on occasion, reports she can have some power in certain situations by aligning with Lilyan.

      e. *Secrets/Myths*: Because they are so open with each other, there are few *secrets*. Aviva does tell Helen secrets and she is left with the awful choice of keeping Aviva's confidence (her power) or telling the parents something they really need to know. Errol will not discuss his family of origin and their religious practices. Any broad or pervasive family *myths* are not identified.

   3. Family Spirituality—Because the father is a clergyman, they were socialized in a religious atmosphere (attending services, parochial schools for several years, confirmation). However, the children state they were not force-fed religion. The parents are liberal in their tolerance of other religious/spiritual viewpoints. Aviva has married two men who are not of her religion. Helen has dated males of different religions (present relationship excluded), but intends to marry a man of the same religion, as she wants to ensure that her religion continues.

C. Family Relationship Map

   1. The family type according to FACES-III was in the mid-range but near "rigidly disengaged" (see Figure 3.4). Family concerns centered around the distance between the parents and their older daughter, which has not been resolved since her marriage to Brian. Figure 8.1 depicts Aviva's family relationships during her two marriages.

II. Cultural Aspects
   Operationalization of variables within the family:

   A. Time—family is present- and future-oriented; time was more family-centered when children were younger but more outward-centered as children became adults

B. Space—there were clear boundaries between the family and outside; parents seemed overinvolved with Aviva and her family

C. Communication—direct, open but often distance was used when there were disagreements

D. Social organization—parents were head of the family unit

E. Biological variations—none were discussed, which presently affected the family members

F. Environmental control—members seemed to be in control of their lives with guidance from their spiritual faith

III. Summary

A. During the initial interview, all family members agreed the main family problem was related to the parents, especially Errol, and Aviva and her family. However, the family did report that Helen played many roles that were beyond her maturity level and assumed responsibility for others' emotional well-being. Helen has struggled to achieve independence because her family was enmeshed, not allowing enough separateness. This problem is resolving. Because the family religion was not forced on Helen, she is struggling with this presently.

B. Family Strengths

1. *Structural strengths* are the family's internal boundaries that have reinforced feelings of belonging to the family unit and their spending time together as a family, such as eating together.

2. *Process strengths* are that members have always communicated the felt love and communication has been open.

3. The family's *religion/spirituality* has always given them a sense of broader community, pride, and tradition.

4. *Health* has been important to the family and there are not many illnesses.

C. Family Problems

1. *Structural problems* are that Aviva was typecast in her "black sheep" role. She had trouble breaking out of it. Helen functioned as mediator and peacemaker, which were roles she should not have had to play at such a young age. All members agreed that Errol has done "too good" a job at keeping everyone "in line."

2. *Process problems* are that the family was too enmeshed and did not allow enough separateness. The parents have become more separated over how to deal with Aviva. Recently, Errol's communication with his mother has become more conflictual. It is unclear to other family members the reason for this and Errol has not discussed this.

3. *Spiritual problems* relate to Aviva's marriages to two men outside of the family religion and, as a result, her children have no firm religious identity. Helen is unsure of the part that religion plays in her life. Although Errol's heritage on his mother's side is Jewish, what part this has played in his life is not clear.

4. *Health* could be more of an issue in terms of health promotion activities.

D. The *family's response* to this initial assessment was very open and all members participated equally. Members allowed other members to air different views that were discussed respectfully among them. Some topics, such as Errol's religious heritage, were not examined in depth, even though he was asked by his children to discuss this.

Internal and external factors (in italics) related to family health: Physically, they were brought up in a safe environment with enough food, clothing, and more-than-adequate shelter. The mother cooked healthy foods. Both parents encouraged exercise and fun. *Mentally,* although the father "has conflicts with his family," he was able to separate himself from these hereditary forces and made a "wonderful husband and father" (family members reported this was largely because of the mother's positive experiences in her family of origin). They had struggles with mental health issues through the years but were not afraid to turn to others for help (these were referred to but not made specific). The family, especially the father, reports that his *spiritual beliefs* are "the mainstay of his existence." Errol being a minister, the family was heavily influenced by sociocultural forces, yet, as these were largely spiritually based, they saw them as positive. Although the family knew much about their *cultural heritage*, the members did not see this as contributing much to their family nor playing a role in family decisions. The family incorporated *hereditary and environmental forces* into its beliefs about wellness. Although earlier there were some reported health problems, some not discussed in detail, there were financial resources to deal with these. The family reports they are avid readers/watchers of the latest health breakthroughs and incorporated some of these into their lifestyle.

IV. Goals/Interventions

A. Goals

At the initial interviews, for the future, the family stated they wanted to continue to deal with their health problems in an open manner. Due to their closeness, they wanted to continue to be involved in each other's lives (regardless of geographic distance) and family members see this as positive. "We help each other out even if there is a strain in our relationship." Although the initial reason for coming to therapy was the father's concern about his oldest daughter, all family members want some resolution of the tension that exists among them and all family members.

B. Interventions

When asked on the initial interview what the family wanted to happen for the family, Helen said she would like to more fully confront past issues/events that had a very negative impact on the family. However, she was not sure if it would be better for their mental and spiritual well-being to just let the past be. After the initial interviews, review of the genogram and ecomap, and discussions with the family, interventions would seem to be focused on unresolved issues between Errol and Aviva. Although the members see their closeness as a resource, more individuation needs to occur with members so that Helen can leave the family without taking the role of the black sheep as her sister did. As the family seems unaware of the influence of their cultural heritage, this can be explored to see if it holds some of the answers regarding spiritual concerns. The distance that has been created between the parents due to conflicts over Aviva need to be addressed.

C. Referrals
    None indicated on initial assessment.

Treatment Plan

The treatment plan flows from the goals stated by the family: (a) maintain or increase openness among all family members, (b) openly discuss health problems, and (c) increase comfort level among all family members over past tensions in the family.

Interventions—The Therapy Process

The complete course of therapy cannot be reviewed here. However, examples of interventions are given based on the theories and concepts referred to earlier in the book (these found in parentheses in the Intervention column of Table 8.1). In order to work constructively with families with a different cultural heritage, clinicians must possess the following skills: self-knowledge skills; assessment skills; therapeutic communication and intervention skills; spiritual skills; case management skills; collaboration and consultation skills; and skills regarding referrals, family support, and resources (Cox, 1995, 1999). These skills are imbedded within and influenced by the cultural context of the clinician and the family. Table 8.1 lists the skills, components for the therapist, and examples of how these skills were used when working with the Belcher family. The theories and concepts discussed earlier in the book, which guided the interventions, are identified with many of the interventions.

Evaluation/Outcomes

Throughout the treatment process, the clinician and family re-evaluated the goals that had been initially set, resulting in new goals being adopted. These new goals related to Errol working on his parental relationship, while Aviva worked on being less conflicted with Mark about the children. Compared to the initial Family Assessment, the family reported that they "felt less tension regarding issues with Aviva and her first marriage." Results of FACES-III showed the family more toward the normal range (see Figure 3.4). When considering treatment goals, the family reported "We have been able to talk about difficult issues from the past." Helen said she now understood why spirituality was so important when considering her father's cultural heritage.

Posttreatment goals were as follow: (a) Errol will call his mother once a month, (b) Judy will talk with Helen about her spirituality, and (c) Errol will see his physician regarding some concerns about his health (these were never specified). The clinician said she was available for consultation if needed. Errol and Judy both wanted to become more knowledgeable about their cultural heritage and how that has affected their family. Therefore, a posttreatment appointment was set for two months.

Table 8.1.
Skills, Therapist Components, and Examples Used with the Belcher Family

Skills	Therapist Components	Intervention Examples
Self-knowledge skills	• Identify and acknowledge their own thoughts, beliefs, feelings, actions, and biases that are influenced by their culture and the family's	• Therapist (T) acknowledged her anxiety over knowing nothing about the family's cultural, questioning culturally competent interventions (Giger and Davidhizar)
	• Aware of his or her own family dynamics to preclude confusing his or her own family of origin issues with those of clients and families	• T has a conflictual, unresolved relationship with her mother and often sides against mothers (Bowen- Family Projection Process- T's family-of-origin)
	• Attend to own health issues with coping skills (i.e., exercise, nurturance, and support from colleagues and friends)	• T has become overwhelmed by work but has not met with colleagues
	• Learn to think "circularly" rather than linearly (as in cause and effect)	• T asked circular question (Tomm): "Errol, how do you think your health problems and your family problems are related? (Triangle of Family Health-physical health) "How do you see what has been happening in your family impacting your work outside the family?" (Triangle of Family Health-environmental factors)
	• Resist constantly the idea to view one family member as "the problem" - have the view of *multipartiality*, the view that all members' ideas are equally valuable and justifiable and all can contribute to the solution of the problem	• T asked circular question (Tomm): "Helen, how has your parents' relationship with Aviva affected your relationship with your sister? (Bowen-triangles) T asked linear question (Tomm): "How did you all manage to stay close to one another as you grew up?" (Olson-cohesion) T asked (Anderson-collaboration): "How did you all work together to find a solution for the family problems/"

Table 8.1.
Continued

Assessment skills	• View systematically interactions within their cultural context, *among* all family members as sources for family problem solving	• T initially asked the parents about the problem (Bowenian approach); next, other adult family members (Olson-communication); and then all members (FACES-III Olson)
	• View family as a collaborative partner in health care problem solving and decision making	• T asked the family their goals for therapy (see Assessment) and then goals became part of the Treatment Plan
	• View all aspects of information gathering as "family-perceived" and "professional-perceived"	• T involved all family members in discussions and shared her view with the family
	• Partnership to clarify discrepant views and to discover fresh alternatives for action (Lapp, Diemert, and Enestvedt, 1993)	• T asked circular question (Tomm): "Aviva, you seem to think your father is unfair while your father thinks you are not attentive to the children's spirituality. What are your ideas?" (Bowen-differentiation) T asked a reflexive question (Tomm) as possible alternative action: "Errol and Aviva, if you began thinking that you had the best interests of the children in mind and *worked together*, what would happen?" (Bowen-emotional cutoff)
Therapeutic communication skills	• Interact simultaneously with all family members with the same amount of respect and nonjudgment	• T: "Aviva, I understand you have been rude to your father at his church; how do you want to handle disagreements now?" (Tomm- reflexive question) (Bowen-differentiation) T: "Errol and Judy, how have you handled your disagreements over Aviva?"(Tomm-linear question) (Bowen-nuclear family emotional system-marital conflict)

(continued)

Table 8.1.
Continued

	• Have beliefs that include: * families are functioning the best that they can and can solve their own problems; strengths exist in all families; parents are doing the best job they can; + no one is the blame for the family problems; and people act in unconstructive ways when protecting and shielding themselves from painful interactions	• T: * "I know that the disagreements in your family have been troubling to you all. I also hear that all of you want this to be different in the future and are all here to solve these past problems." (Olson-flexibility) (Anderson-collaboration) + "The way I am thinking about what has happened is that all have been a part, even though Errol, for you, the concern is with Aviva and the children." (Bowen-differentiation)
	• Attend to interactions *between and among* members of the system rather than the actions of one individual	• T observes the family discussing Aviva's first marriage (Process-separateness/ connectedness)
Intervention skills	• Have a working knowledge of families, systems, culture, and family theories as a basis for culturally competent interventions	• T asks the family to teach her about their cultural heritage, esp. Errol concerning communication about spirituality (Giger and Davidhizar-communication)
	• Intervene based on information received from the client and family within their cultural context and meaning system	• T: "Judy, how were things organized in your family around religious practices?" (Tomm-linear question) (Giger and Davidhizar-social organization)
	• Interview is a circular phenomenon between the therapist, client, and family (Wright and Leahey, 1994)	• As Aviva teaches the T about her relationship with Mark, the T asks the father what he understands differently (moving more toward flexibility based on FACES-III)
	• Have knowledge of various teaching strategies and learning principals as all families do not learn information in the same way	• T asks family members how they best like to learn new information

Table 8.1.
Continued

Spiritual skills	• Aware of facilitative attitudes (i.e., tolerance, forgiveness, nonreactiveness, encouragement, and hopefulness) rooted in a spiritual dimension (Carson, 1989) • Intervene effectively with family members by entering into a relationship, becoming a companion in his or her journey, and sharing the person's emotions such as pain, anger, or sadness (H. Anderson, 1997; Carson, 1989)	• T and Judy discuss how she has been hopeful for Aviva where as Errol has been upset with her (Triangle of Family Health-spirituality) • T shares Aviva's pain and agony over her disappointing her father in her second divorce from Mark while the T empathizes with Helen over her lack of spiritual direction (Triangle of Family Health-spirituality) T asks: "Errol, in the family you grew up in, what say did you have in your own spiritual growth?" (Tomm-linear question) (Giger and Davidhizar-environmental control) T asks: "Errol and Avivia, what has it meant to you two to be at such odds with each other over the children?" (Anderson-meaning) (Hill-definition of events)
Case management skills	• View aspects within the family as well as outside the family (i.e., the community, schools, churches, and governments) • Assist families in dealing with the many problems they face • Provide crisis intervention when necessary	• Family discusses how disagreements within the family have affected their religious life as a family • T can serve as an intermediary when dealing with other agencies • Although no crisis exists now, T would be available to meet with the family, being open to meeting in their home if necessary (Bowen-lowering anxiety within the system)

(continued)

Table 8.1.
Continued

Collaboration and consultation skills	• Work effectively as a peer with colleagues in assisting families and meeting family goals	• Consult with Aviva's first therapist when appropriate (Anderson-collaboration)
	• Work toward family outcomes with other disciplines (i.e., other health professionals, school boards, and advisory boards)	• Work with school boards to provide parenting classes in the schools
	• Work with legislators on family issues	• Work for new laws (i.e., Florida's Marriage Preparations and Preservation Act of 1998) (Bowen-societal regression) Promote universal access to health care
	• Maintain attention to collaborative values (McDaniel and Campbell, 1996)	• Focus primarily on capacities as opposed to deficits; value interdependency
	• Become accountable for the use of resources	• Track statistics and outcomes
Referrals, family support, and resources skills	• Support families as they enter the desired system for assistance	• Empower family to involve extended family members in resolution of family problems Assist family with identifying resources and coping mechanisms useful to the family in stressful situations (Hill-resources)

References

After 260 grim days, silence. (2002, May 31). *Portland Press Herald*, p. 1A.

Ahrons, C. (1980, November). Redefining the divorced family. A conceptual framework. *Social Work*, 437–441.

Ahrons, C. (1998). Divorce: An unscheduled family transition. In B. Carter & M. McGoldrick (Eds.), *The expanded family life cycle: Individual, family, and social perspectives* (3rd ed., pp. 381–398). Boston: Allyn & Bacon.

Ahrons, C., & Rodgers, R. (1987). *Divorced families: A multidisciplinary developmental view*. New York: Norton.

Aldous, J. (1978). *Family careers: Developmental change in families*. New York: Wiley.

Aldous, J. (1996). *Family careers: Rethinking the developmental perspective*. Thousand Oaks, CA: Sage.

American Association for Marriage & Family Therapy (AAMFT). (2001, February/March). *Are MFTs ready for the genomic era?* Washington, DC: Author.

American Nurses Association. (2001). Position statement: Cultural diversity in nursing practice (online). Available: http://www.nursingworld.org/readroom/position/ethics/etcldv.htm

American Psychiatric Association (APA). (2000a). *Diagnostic and statistical manual of mental disorders-Fourth Edition-Text Revision*. Washington, DC: Author.

American Psychiatric Association. (July 26, 2000b). Major depressive disorder: A patient and family guide (online). Available: http://www.psych.org/clin_res./MajorDepression.pdf

American Psychiatric Association (July 26, 2000c). Major depressive disorder: A patient and family guide (online). Available: http://www.psych.org/clin_res./Delirium.pdf

Ames, K. (1992). Domesticated bliss: New laws are making it official for gay and live-in couples. *Newsweek, 40*, 46–47.

Andersen, T. (1987). The reflecting team: Dialogue and metadialogue in clinical work. *Family Process, 26*, 415–428.

Anderson, H. (Speaker). (1991a). *A collective language systems approach to therapy* (Video No. V521). Washington, DC: The American Association for Marriage and Family Therapy.

Anderson, H. (Speaker). (1991b). *Creating a language of change* (Video No. V308). Washington, DC: The American Association for Marriage and Family Therapy.

Anderson, H. (1997). *Conversation, language, and possibilities*. New York: Basic Books.

Anderson, H., & Goolishian, H. (1988). Human systems as linguistic systems: Prelim-
inary and evolving ideas about the implications for clinical theory. *Family Process, 27*(4), 371–393.

Anderson, K., & Tomlinson, P. (1992). The family health system as an emerging par-
adigmatic view for nursing. *Image: Journal of Nursing Scholarship, 24*, 57–63.

Aneshensel, C., Pearlin, L., Mullan, J., Zarit, S., & Whitlatch, C. (1995). *Profiles in
caregiving: The unexpected career*. San Diego: Academic Press.

Arredondo, P., Toporek, R., Brown, S., Jones, J., Locke, D., Sanchez, J., & Stadler, H.
(1996). Operationalization of the multicutural counseling competencies. *Journal
of Multicultural Counseling and Development, 24*, 42–78.

Artinian, N. (1994). Selecting a model to guide family assessment. *Dimensions of Critical Care Nursing, 14*(1), 4–16.

Bateson, G. (1972). *Steps to an ecology of mind*. New York: Ballantine Books.

Bateson, G. (1979). *Mind and nature: A necessary unity*. New York: Bantam Books.

Barbell, K. (1997). *Foster care today: A briefing paper*. Washington, DC: Child Welfare
League of America.

Bata, E., & Power, P. (1995). Facilitating health care decisions within aging families. In
G. Smith, S. Tobin, E. Robertson, T. Chabo, & P. Power (Eds.), *Strengthening
aging families* (pp. 143–157). Thousand Oaks, CA: Sage.

Beavers, W. (1977). *Psychotherapy and growth: A family systems perspective*. New
York: Brunner/Mazel.

Beavers, W., & Hampson, R. (1990). *Successful families: Assessment and Intervention*.
New York: W. W. Norton.

Beavers, W., Hampson, R., & Hulgus, Y. (1990). *Manual: Beavers systems model of
family assessment*. Dallas: Southwest Family Institute.

Berry, J., Poortinga, Y., Segall, M., & Dansen, P. (1992). *Cross-cultural psychology:
Research and applications*. New York: Cambridge University Press.

Blechman, E., & McEnroe, M. (1985). Effective family problem solving. *Child Development, 56*, 429–437.

Berger, R. (1998). *Stepfamilies: A multidimensional perspective*. Binghamton, NY:
Haworth Press.

Biegel, D., Sales, E., & Schulz, R. (1991). *Family caregiving in chronic illness*. Newbury
Park, CA: Sage.

Blazer, D. G. (1984). Evaluating the family of the elderly patient. In D. Blazer & I.
Seigler (Eds.), *A Family Approach to Health Care in the Elderly* (pp. 13–32).
Menlo Park, CA: Addison-Wesley.

Blazer, D. G. (1996). The psychiatric interview of the geriatric patient. In E. Busse & D.
Blazer (Eds.), *Textbook of geriatric psychiatry* (2nd ed., pp. 175–209). Washington, DC: American Psychiatric Press.

Bomar, P. (Ed.). (1989). *Nurses and family health promotion: Concepts assessment, and
intervention*. Philadelphia: W. B. Saunders.

Bomar, P. (Ed.) (1996). Nurses and family health promotion: Concepts assessment, and
intervention (2nd ed.). Philadelphia: Saunders.

Bond, M. (1994). Into the heart of collectivism: A personal and scientific journey. In U.
Kim, H. Triandis, C. Kagitcibasi, S. Choi, & G. Yoon (Eds.), *Individualism and
collectivism: Theory, method and applications* (pp. 66–76). Thousand Oaks, CA:
Sage.

Bowen, M. (1978). *Family therapy in clinical practice*. New York: Jason Aronson.

Bradshaw, J. (1988). *Bradshaw on the family*. Deefield Beach, FL: Health Communications.

Bray, J. (1995). Assessment of family health and distress: An intergenerational-systems perspective. In J. C. Conoley & E. Werth (Eds.), *Family assessment* (pp. 125–140). Lincoln: Buros Institute of Measurement, University of Nebraska.

Breunlin, D. Schwartz, R. Kune-Karrer, B. (1992). *Meta Frameworks: L Ramscending the models of family therapy*. San Francisco: Jossey-Bass.

Brody, E. (1985). Parent care as a normative family stress. *Gerontologist, 25*, 19–29.

Brody, E. (1990). *Women in the middle: Their parent care years*. New York: Springer.

Brody, E. (1995). Prospects for family caregiving: Response to change, continuity, and diversity. In R. A. Kane & J. D. Penrod (Eds.), *Family caregiving in an aging society: Policy perspectives* (pp. 15–28). Thousand Oaks, CA: Sage.

Brody, E., Litvin, S., Kleben, M., & Hoffman, C. (1990, November). *Differential effects of daughters' marital status on their parent care experience*. Paper presented at the 43rd annual meeting of the Gerontological Society of America, Boston, MA.

Bulger, M., Wandersman, A., & Goldman, C. (1993). Burdens and gratifications of caregiving: Appraisal of parental care of adults with schizophrenia. *American Journal of Orthopsychiatry, 64*, 255–265.

Bumpass, L., Sweet, S., & Cherlin, A. (1991). The role of cohabitation in declining rates of marriage. *Journal of Marriage and the Family, 53*, 913–927.

Butz, M. (1997). *Chaos and complexity*. Washington, DC: Taylor & Francis.

Carruth, A. (1996). Development and testing of the Caregiver Reciprocity Scale. *Nursing Research, 45*(2), 92–97.

Carson, V. (1989). *Spiritual dimensions of nursing practice*. Philadelphia: Saunders.

Carter, B., & McGoldrick, M. (Eds.). (1989). *The changing family life cycle: A framework for family therapy* (2nd ed., p. 22). New York: Gardner Press.

Carter, B., & McGoldrick, M. (1999). The divorce cycle: A major variation in the American family life cycle. In B. Carter & M. McGoldrick (Eds.), *The expanded family life cycle: Individual, family & social perspectives* (3rd ed., pp. 373–380). Boston: Allyn & Bacon.

Chu, J. (1992). The therapeutic roller coaster: Dilemmas in the treatment of childhood abuse survivors. *Journal of Psychotherapy Practice and Research, 1*, 351–370.

Clarkin, J., Frances, A., & Moodie, J. (1979). Selection criteria for family therapy. *Family Process, 18*, 391–404.

Cockerham, W. (1987). *Medical sociology* (2nd ed.). Englewood Cliffs, NJ: Prentice-Hall.

Coe, R. (1970). *Sociology of medicine*. New York: McGraw-Hill.

Constantine, M., Juby, H., & Liang, J. (2001). Examining multicultural counseling competence and race-related attitudes among white marital and family therapists. *Journal of Marital and Family Therapy, 27*(3), 353–362.

Corcoran, K., & Fisher, J. (1987). *Measures for clinical practice*. New York: Free Press.

Coupland, S., Serovich, J., & Glenn, J. (1995). Reliability in constructing genograms: A study among marriage and family therapy doctoral students. *Journal of Marital and Family Therapy, 21*(3), 251–263.

Cox, R. P. (1993). The human/animal bond as a correlate of family functioning. *Clinical Nursing Research, 2*(2), 224–231.

Cox, R. P. (1994). Systemic circularity: Working with individuals for family level change. *Journal of Psychosocial Nursing and Mental Health Services, 32*(7), 33–39.

Cox, R. P. (1995). Working with the family. In N. Keltner, L. Schwecke, & C. Bostrom (Eds.), *Psychiatric nursing* (2nd ed., pp. 147–162). St. Louis, MO: Mosby.

Cox, R. P. (1997). Family health care delivery for the 21st century. *Journal of Obstetric, Gynecologic, and Neonatal Nursing, 26*(1), 109–118.

Cox, R. P. (1999). Working with the family. In N. Keltner, L. Schwecke, & C. Bostrom (Eds.), *Psychiatric nursing* (3rd ed., pp. 181–198). St. Louis, MO: Mosby.

Cox, R. P. (in press). Theory-based family problem-solving interventions. *Clinical Excellence for Nurse Practitioners.*

Cox, R. P., & Davis, L. L. (1993). Social constructivist approaches for brief, episodic, problem-focused family encounters. *Nurse Practitioner, 18*(8), 45–49.

Cox, R. P., & Davis, L. L. (1999). Family problem-solving: Measuring the elusive concept. *Journal of Family Nursing, 5*(3), 332–360.

Coyle, S. M. (1999). *Review of the soul in distress: What every pastoral counselor should know about emotional and mental illness.* By Richard Roukema, MD. (online). Available: http://www.oates.org/journal/pub/vol-02-99/reviews/soul_in_distress. html

Curran, D. (1983). *Traits of a healthy family.* San Francisco: Harper & Row.

Curran, D. (1985). *Stress and the healthy family.* San Francisco: Harper & Row.

Dana, R. (1993). *Multicultural assessment perspectives for professional psychology.* Boston: Allyn & Bacon.

Danielson, C., Hamel-Bissell, B., & Winstead-Fry, P. (1993). *Families, health, & illness.* St. Louis, MO: Mosby.

Davis L. L., & Cox, R. P. (1995). Using interventive questions to empower family decision making. *Dimensions of Critical Care Nursing, 14*(1), 48–55.

DeFrain, J., & Stinnett, N. (1992). Building on the inherent strengths of families: A positive approach for family psychologists and counselors. *Topics in Family Psychology and Counseling, 1*, 15–26.

Degazon, C. (1996). Cultural diversity and community health nursing practice. In M. Stanhope & J. Lancaster, *Community health nursing: Promoting health of aggregates, families, and individuals* (4th ed., pp. 117–134). St. Louis, MO: Mosby.

de Jonghe, F., Kool, S., van Aalst, G., Dekker J., & Peen J. (2001). Combining psychotherapy and antidepressants in the treatment of depression. *Journal of Affective Disorders, 64*(2–3), 217–229.

de la Torre, A. (1993, March 31). Access is vital in health care reform. *Los Angles Times,* p. B7.

DeMaria, R., Weeks, G., & Hof, L. (1999). *Focused genograms.* Philadelphia: Bruner/ Mazel.

Dicks, H. (1967). *Marital tensions.* London: Routledge & Kegan Paul.

Dienhart, A., & Avis, J. (1994). Working with men in family therapy: An exploratory study. *Journal of Marital and Family Therapy, 20*(4), 397–417.

Divan, D. (1989). Letter to the editor. *New England Journal of Medicine, 321*(4), 259.

Doherty, W. (1985). Family intervention in health care. *Family Relations, 34*, 129–137.

Doherty, W., & Campbell, T. (1988). *Families and health.* Newbury Park, CA: Sage.

Doherty, W., & McCubbin, H. (1985). Families and health care: An emerging arena of theory, research and clinical interventions. *Family Relations, 34*, 5–11.

Doornbos, M. (1997). The problems and coping methods of caregivers of young adults with mental illness. *Journal of Psychosocial Nursing and Mental Health Services, 35*(9), 22–26.

Dozier, R., Hicks, M., Cornille, T., & Peterson, G. (1998). The effect of Tomm's questioning style on therapeutic alliance: An analog study. *Family Process 37*(2), 189–200.

Duvall, E. (1971). *Family development* (4th ed.). Philadelphia: J. B. Lippincott.

Duvall, E. (1977). *Marriage and family development* (5th ed.). Philadelphia: Lippincott.

Duvall, E., & Miller, B. (1985). *Marriage and family development* (6th ed.). New York: Harper & Row.

Dwyer, J., & Coward, R. (1991). A multivariate comparison of the involvement of adult sons versus daughters in the care of impaired parents. *Journal of Gerontology, 46*, S259–269.

Ebersole, P., & Hess, P. (Eds.). (1994). *Toward healthy aging human needs and nursing response* (4th ed.). St. Louis: Mosby-Year Book.

Empirically validated and evidence based treatments. (2000, October/November). *Family Therapy News,* 22–23.

Epstein, N., Bishop, D., & Baldwin, L. (1982). McMaster model of family functioning: A view of the normal family. In F. Walsh (Ed.), *Normal family processes* (pp. 115–141). New York: Guilford.

Epstein, N., Baldwin, L., & Bishop, D. (1983). The McMaster Family Assessment Device. *Journal of Martial and Family Therapy, 9*, 171–180.

Fawcett, J. (1989). *Analysis and evaluation of conceptual model of nursing* (2nd ed.). Philadelphia: Davis.

Fein, E. (1998, October 24). Secrecy and stigma no longer clouding adoptions. *The New York Times,* Section 1, p. 1.

Finley, N. (1989). Theories of family labor as applied to gender differences in caregiving for elderly parents. *Journal of Marriage and the Family, 51*(1), 79–86.

Fisher, L. (1976). Dimensions of family assessment: A critical review. *Journal of Marriage and Family Counseling, 2*, 367–382.

Foley, V., & Everett, C. (Eds.). (1981). *Family therapy glossary.* (Available from the American Association for Marriage and Family Therapy, 1100 17th St. NW 10th Floor, Washington, DC 20036).

Friedemann, M. (1989). Closing the gap between grand theory and mental health practice with families. Part 1. *Archives of Psychiatric Nursing, III (February),* 10–19.

Friedman, M. (1986). *Family nursing: Theory and assessment* (2nd ed.). Norwalk, CT: Appleton-Century-Crofts.

Friedman, M. (1998). *Family nursing: Theory and assessment* (4th ed.). Stamford, CT: Appleton-Century-Crofts.

Fulmer, R. (1989). Lower-income and professional families: A comparison of structure and life cycle process. In B. Carter & M. McGoldrick (Eds.), *The changing family life cycle* (pp. 545–578). New York: Gardner Press.

Giger, J., & Davidhizar, R. (1995). *Transcultural nursing—Assessment and intervention.* St. Louis: Mosby.

Gilliss, C. (1991). Family nursing research: theory and practice. *Image, 23*(1), 19–24.

Gilliss, C. (1993). Family nursing research, theory, and practice. In G. D. Wegner & R. J. Alexander (Eds.), *Readings in family nursing* (pp. 34–42). Philadelphia: Lippincott.

Gilliss, C., & Davis, L. (1993). Does family intervention make a difference? An integrative review and meta-analysis. In S. Feetham, S. Meister, J. Bell, & C. Gilliss

(Eds.), *The nursing of families: Theory/research/education/practice* (pp. 259–265). Newbury Park, CA: Sage.

Goldenberg, I., & Goldenberg, H. (1991). *Family therapy—An overview* (3rd ed.). Pacific Grove, CA: Brooks/Cole.

Goldenberg, H., & Goldenberg, I. (1998). *Counseling today's family* (3rd ed.). Pacific Grove, CA: Brooks/Cole.

Goldstein, M. (1985). Family factors that antedate the onset of schizophrenia and related disorders: The results of a fifteen-year prospective longitudinal study. *Acta Psychiatrica Scandinavia, 319* (Suppl.), 7–18.

Goldstein, M., & Strachan, A. (1987). The family and schizophrenia. In T. Jacob (Ed.), *Family interactions and psychopathology* (pp. 481–504). New York: Plenum.

Gonzalez, R. (1997). Postmodern supervision: A mulitcultural perspective. In D. B. Pope-Davis & H. K. Coleman (Eds.), *Multicultural counseling competencies: Assessment, education and training, and supervision* (pp. 350–386). Thousand Oaks, CA: Sage.

Gore, S., & Mangione, T. (1983). Social roles, sex roles, and psychological distress. *Journal of Health and Social Behavior, 24,* 300–312.

Gove, W., Hughes, M., & Style, C. (1983). Does marriage have positive effects on the psychological well-being of the individual? *Journal of Health and Social Behavior, 24,* 122–131.

Green, R., Kolevzon, M., & Vosler, N. (1985). The Beavers-Timberlawn Model of Family Competence and the Circumplex Model of Family-Adapability and Cohesion: Separate but equal? *Family Process, 24,* 385–398.

Greenberg, J., Greenley, J., McKee, D., Brown, R., & Griffin-Francell, C. (1993). Mothers caring for an adult child with schizophrenia: The effects of subjective burden on maternal health. *Family Relations, 42,* 205–211.

Griffin-Francell, C. (1993). Psychiatric nurses must be held accountable for their actions. *Journal of Psychosocial Nursing and Mental Health Services, 31*(10), 5–12.

Grossman, D. (1996). Cultural dimensions in home health nursing. *American Journal of Nursing, 96*(7), 33–36.

Grotevant, H. (1989). The role of theory in guiding family assessment. *Journal of Family Psychology, 3*(2), 104–117.

Grotevant, H., & Carlson, C. (1989). *Family assessment: A guide to methods and measures.* New York: Guilford Press.

Grothaus, K. (1996). Family dynamics and family therapy with Mexican Americans. *Journal of Psychosocial Nursing, 34*(2), 31–37.

Hajal, F., & Rosenberg, E. (1991). The family life cycle in adoptive families. *American Journal of Orthopsychiatry, 61*(1), 78–85.

Hanson, S. (2001). *Family health care nursing: theory, practice, and research* (2nd ed.). Philadelphia, PA: Davis.

Hanson, S., & Boyd, S. (1996). *Family health care nursing: theory, practice, and research.* Philadelphia, PA: Davis.

Hardy, K., & Laszloffy, T. (1995). The cultural genogram: Key to training culturally competent family therapists. *Journal of Marital and Family Therapy, 21*(3), 227–237.

Harper, M. (1995). An overview of mental health. In M. Hogstel (Ed.), *Geropsychiatric nursing* (2nd ed.). St. Louis: Mosby-Year Book.

Hartman, A. (1996). Social policy as a context for lesbian and gay families. The political is personal. In J. Laird & R-J. Green (Eds.), *Lesbian and gays in couples and families. A handbook for therapists* (pp. 69–85). San Francisco: Jossey-Bass.

Harvath, T., Stewart, B., & Archibold, P. (1994, May 25–28). *Third International Family Nursing Conference, Program and Abstracts*. Montreal, Canada.

Hatfield, A., & Letley, H. (1993). *Surviving mental illness: Stress, coping, and adaption*. New York: Guilford.

Healy, J., Malley, J., & Stewart, A. (1990). Children and their fathers after parental separation. *American Journal of Orthopsychiatry, 60*(4), 531–543.

Helman, C. (1990). *Culture, health and illness: An introduction for health professionals*. London: Wright.

Hellwig, K. (1993). Psychiatric home care nursing: Managing patients in the community setting. *Journal of Psychosocial Nursing and Mental Health Services, 31*(12), 21–27.

Helmeke, K., & Prouty, A. (2001). Do we really understand? An experimental exercise for training family therapists. *Journal of Marital and Family Therapy, 27*(4), 535–544.

Heppner, P., Cook, S., Strozier, A., & Heppner, M. (1991). An investigation of coping styles and gener differences with farmers in career transition. *Journal of Counseling Psychology, 38*, 167–174.

Herman, J., Perry, J., & van der Kolk, B. (1989). Childhood trauma in borderline personality disorder. *American Journal of Psychiatry, 146*, 490–495.

Hetherington, E., Law, T., & O'Connor, T. (1993). DIVORCE: Challenges, changes, and new changes. In F. Walsh (Ed.), *Normal family processes* (2nd ed., pp. 208–234). New York: Guilford.

Hill, R. (1949). *Families under stress*. New York: Harper & Row.

Hill, R. (1958). Social stresses on the family: Generic features of families under stress. *Social Casework, 39*, 139–150.

Hill, R. (1965). *Challenges and resources for family development. Family mobility in our dynamic society*. Ames, IA: Iowa State University.

Hill, R. (1986). Life cycle stages for types of single parent families: Of family development theory. *Family Relations, 35*(1), 19–29.

Hines, P. (1988). The family life cycle of poor black families. In B. Carter & M. McGoldrick (Eds.), *The changing life cycle* (pp. 513–544). New York: Gardner.

Horowitz, A. (1985). Family caregiving to the frail elderly. In C. Eisdorder, P. Lawton, & G. Maddox (Eds.), *Annual review of gerontology and geriatrics*, (Vol. 5, pp. 194–246). New York: Springer.

Horwitz, S., Owens, P., & Simms, M. (2000). Specialized assessments for children in foster care. *Pediatrics, 106*(1), 59–66.

Inouye, J. (1999). Asian American health and disease: an overview of the issues. In R. Huff & M. Kline (Eds.), *Promoting health in multicultural populations: A handbook for practitioners* (pp. 337–356). Thousand Oaks, CA: Sage.

Joyner, D., & Swenson, D. (1993). Community level interventions afer a disaster. In C. F. Saylor (Ed.), *Children and disasters* (pp. 211–232). New York: Plenum Press.

Kagitcibasi, C. (1996). *Family and human development across cultures*. Mahwah, NJ: Erlbaum.

Kahana, E., Kahana, B., Johnson, J., Hammand, R., & Kercher, K. (1994). Developmental challenges and family caregiving: Bridging concepts and research. In E. Kahana,

D. Biegel, & M. Wykle (Eds.), *Family caregiving across the life span* (pp. 3–42). Thousand Oaks, CA: Sage.

Kandel, D., Davies, M., & Raveis, V. (1985). The stressfulness of daily social roles for women: Marital, occupational, and household roles. *Journal of Health and Social Behavior, 26*, 64–78.

Karon, B. (1994). Is there really a schizophrenogenic parent? *Psychoanalytic Psychology, 11*, 47–61.

Keefe, S. (1981). Folk medicine among Mexican-Americans: Cultural persistence, change and displacement. *Hispanic Journal of Behavior Science, 3*, 41–48.

Kelly, A. (1978). *Evaluating and improving family health: The holistic health handbook.* Berkeley, CA: And/Or Press.

Keltner, N. (2000a). Neuroreceptor function and psychopharmacologic response. *Issues in Mental Health Nursing, 21*, 31–50.

Keltner, N. (2000b). Mechanisms of antidepressant action: In brief. *Perspectives in Psychiatric Care, 36*, 69–71.

Keltner, N., Coffeen, H., & Johnson, J. (2000). Atypical antipsychotic drugs: Part II. *Perspectives in Psychiatric Care, 36*, 139–140.

Keltner, N., & Folks, D. (2001). *Psychotropic drugs.* St. Louis, MO: Mosby.

Keltner, N., Hogan, B., & Guy, D. (2001). Dopaminergic and serotonergic receptor function in the CNS. *Perspectives in Psychiatric Care, 37*, 65–72.

Keltner, N., Hogan, B., Knight, T., & Royals, L. (in press). Adrenergic, cholingergic, GABAergic, and glutaminergic function in the CNS. *Perspectives in Psychiatric Care.*

Keltner, N., Schwecke, L. & Bostrom, C. (in press). *Psychiatric nursing* (4th ed.). St. Louis, MO: Mosby.

Keltner, N., Zielinski, A., & Hardin, M. (2001). Drugs used for cognitive symptoms of Alzheimer's Disease. *Perspectives in Psychiatric Care, 37*, 31–34.

Kerr, M. (1981). Family systems theory and therapy. In A. Gurman & D. Kniskern (Eds.), *Handbook of family therapy* (1st ed., pp. 226–264). New York: Brunner/Mazel.

Kerr, M., & Bowen, M. (1988). *Family evaluation: An approach based on Bowen theory.* New York: Norton.

Klein, D., & White, J. (1996). *Family theories: An introduction.* Thousand Oaks, CA: Sage.

Kliman, J. (1998). Social class as a relationship: Implications for family therapy. In M. McGoldrick (Ed.), *Re-visioning family therapy: Race, culture, and gender in clinical practice* (pp. 50–61). New York: Guilford.

Knudson-Martin, C. (1997). The politics of gender in family therapy. *Journal of Marital and Family Therapy, 23*(4), 421–437.

Koontz, E., Cox, D., & Hasting, S. (1991). Implementing a short-term family support group. *Journal of Psychosocial Nursing and Mental Health Services, 29*(5), 5–11.

Kramer, J., & Conoley, J., 1992. *The eleventh mental measurements yearbook* (pp. 699–701). Lincoln: University of Nebraska Press.

Kuehl, B. (1995). The solution-oriented genogram: A collaborative approach. *Journal of Marital and Family Therapy, 21*(3), 239–250.

Kumpfer, K., & Kaftarian, S. (2000). Bridging the gap between family-focused research and substance abuse prevention practice: Preface. *The Journal of Primary Prevention, 21*, 169–183.

Laird, J. (1993). Lesbian and gay families. In F. M. Walsh (Ed.), *Normal family process* (2nd ed., pp. 282–328). New York: Norton.

Landau-Stanton, J. (1993). *AIDS, health and mental health: A primary sourcebook.* New York: Brunner/Mazel.

Landy, S., & Munro, S. (1998). Shared parenting: Assessing the success of a foster parent program aimed at family reunification. *Child Abuse & Neglect, 22*(4), 305–318.

Lapp, C., Diemert, C., & Enestvedt, R. (1993). Family-based practice: Discussion of a tool merging assessment with intervention. In G. Wegner & R. Alexander (Eds.), *Readings in family nursing* (pp. 309–316). Philadelphia: Lippincott.

Lee, G. (1982). *Family structure and interaction—A comparative analysis.* Minneapolis: University of Minnesota Press.

Lee, P., & Estes, C. (1997). *The nation's health* (5th ed.). Sudbury, MA: Jones & Bartlett.

Lehne, R. (2001). *Pharmacology for nursing care.* Philadelphia, PA: Saunders.

Leslie, L., Landsverk, J., Ezzet-Lofstrom, J., Slymen, D., & Garland, A. (2000). Children in foster care: Factors influencing outpatient mental health service use. *Child Abuse & Neglect, 24*(4), 465–476.

Lewis, J., Beavers, W., Gossett, J., & Philips, V. (1976). *No single thread. Psychological health in family systems.* New York: Brunner/Mazel.

Liss, L. (1987). Families and the law. In M. Sussman & S. Steinmetz (Ed.), *Handbook of marriage and family* (pp. 767–794). New York: Plenum Press.

Litman, T. (1974). *Health and the family: A three generation study.* Washington, DC: Division of Community Health Services and Medical Care Administration, U.S. Public Health Service.

Lukoff, D., Snyer, D., Ventura, J., & Neuchterlein, D. (1984). Life events, familial stress, and coping in the developmental course of schizophrenia. *Schizophrenia Bulletin, 10,* 258–292.

Maranatha Christian Journal. (2000, March 17). *Gay "Civil Union" passes Vermont House.* Retrieved January 19, 2001 (online). Available: http://www.mcjonline.com/news/oo/20000317c.htm

Marriage Project-Hawaii (1999, May 18). *What is the scope of couples' rights as "Reciprocal Beneficiaries" in Hawaii?* Retrieved December 19, 2001 (online). Available: Marriage Project-Hawaii Web Site: http://members.tripod.com/~MPHAWAII/index3.html

Maturana, H. (1978). The biology of language: The epistimology of reality. In G. Miller & E. Lenneberg (Eds.), *Psychology and biology of language and thought* (pp. 27–63). New York: Academic Press.

Maturana, H., & Varela , R. (1980). *The tree of knowledge.* Boston: New Science Library, Shambhala.

Maturer, H., & Hill, R. (1983). Critical transitions over the family life span: Theory and research. *Marriage and Family Therapy Review 6*(1–2), 39–60.

McCarty, K. (1997, January 27). *Pending adoption legislation—California 1997–1998 Session.* Retrieved December 19, 2001 (online). Available: http://www.webcom/~kmc/adoption/law/ca/pending

McCubbin, M., & McCubbin, H. (1993). Families coping with illness: The resilence model of family stress adjustment and adaptation. In C. B. Danielson, B. Hamel-Bissell, & P. Winstead-Frye (Eds.), *Families in health and illness* (pp. 21–63). St. Louis, MO: Mosby.

McCubbin, M., McCubbin, H., & Thompson, A. (1988). Family problem solving communication. In H. McCubbin, A. Thompson, & M. McCubbin (1996), *Family assessment: Resiliency, coping and adaptation—Inventories for research and practice* (pp. 639–686). Madison: University of Wisconsin System.

McCubbin, H., Olson, D., & Larsen, A. (1981). Family crisis oriented personal scales. In H. McCubbin, A. Thompson, & M. McCubbin (1996), *Family assessment: Resiliency, coping and adaptation—Inventories for research and practice* (pp. 455–507). Madison: University of Wisconsin System.

McCullough, C., Wilson, N., Teasdale, T., Kolpakchi, A., & Skelly, J. (1993). Mapping personal, familial, and professional values in long-term care decisions. *The Gerontologist, 33*(3), 324–332.

McDaniel, S., & Campbell, T. (1996). Training for collaborative family health care. *Families, Systems, & Health, 14*(2), 147–150.

McGoldrick, M., & Carter, E. (1982). The family life cycle. In F. Walsh (Ed.), *Normal family processes* (pp. 167–195). New York: Guilford.

McGoldrick, M. (1996). Foreword. In J. Laird & R-J. Green (Eds.), *Lesbian and gays in couples and families. A handbook for therapists* (p. xi). San Francisco: Jossey-Bass.

McGoldrick, M., & Gerson, R. (1985). *Genograms in family assessment.* New York: Norton.

McGoldrick, M., Heiman, M., & Carter, B. (1993). The changing family life cycle. In F. Walsh (Ed.), *Normal family processes* (2nd ed., pp. 405–443). New York: Guilford.

McLanahan, S., & Adams, J. (1987). Parenthood and psychological well being. *Annual Review of Sociology, 13*, 237–257.

Mederer, H., & Hill, R. (1983). Critical transitions over the family life span. Theory and research. *Marriage and Family Review, 6 (1/2)*, 39–60.

Miller, J. (1990). Use of traditional health care by Korean immigrants to the United States. *Sociology and Social Research, 75*(1), 38–48.

Miller, I., Kabacoff, R., Epstein, N., Bishop, D., Keitner, G., Baldwin, L. & vander Spuy, H. (1994). The development of a clinical rating scale for the McMaster Model of Family Functioning. *Family Process, 33*(1), 53–69.

Mills, D. (1984). A model for stepfamily development. *Family Relations, 33*, 365–372.

Mirowsky, J., & Ross, C. (1989). *Social causes of psychological distress.* New York: Aline-de Grader.

Murata, J. (1994). Family stress, social support, violence and son's behavior. *Western Journal of Nursing Research, 16*, 154–168.

Murdock, G. (1949). *Social structure.* New York: The Free Press.

Neal, M., Chapman, N., Ingersoll-Dayton, B., & Emlen A. (1993). *Balancing work and caregiving for children, adults, and elders.* Thousand Oaks, CA: Sage.

Newman, B. (1983). Family interventions using the Betty Newman health-care system model. In I. W. Clements & F. B. Roberts (Eds.), *Family health: A theoretical approach in nursing care* (pp. 239–254). New York: Wiley.

Nichols, W., & Everett, C. (1986). *Systemic family therapy—An integrative approach.* New York: Guilford.

Nye, I. (1979). Choice, exchange, and the family. In W. Burr, R. Hill, I. Nye, & I. Reiss (Eds.), *Contemporary theories about the family* (Vol. 2, pp. 1–41). New York: The Free Press.

O'Hanlon, W., & Weiner-Davis, M. (1989). *In search of solutions*. New York: Norton.

Olson, D. (1993). Circumplex model of marital and family systems. In F. Walsh (Ed.), *Normal family processes* (pp. 104–137). New York/London: Guilford.

Olson, D., & Tiesel, J. (1991, April). *FACES III: Linear scoring & interpretation*. St. Paul: Family Social Science, University of Minnesota.

Olson, D. (1990). *Clinical rating scale for Circumplex Model*. St. Paul: Family Social Science, University of Minnesota.

Olson, D., McCubbin, H., Barnes, H., Larsen, A., Masan, M., & Wilson, M. (Eds.). (1986). *Family inventories*. St. Paul: Family Social Science, University of Minnesota.

Olson, D., Portner, J., & Lavee, Y. (1985). *FACES III*. St. Paul: Family Social Science, University of Minnesota.

Paniagua, F. (1994). *Assessing and treating culturally diverse clients*. Thousand Oaks, CA: Sage.

Pearsall, P. (1990). *The power of the family: Strength, comfort, and healing*. New York: Doubleday.

Peck, J., & Manocharian, J. (1988). Divorce in the changing family life cycle. In B. Carter & M. McGoldrick (Eds.), *The changing family life cycle* (pp. 335–369). New York: Gardner.

Pedersen, P. (1991a). Multiculturalism as a fourth force in counseling (Special issue). *Journal of Counseling and Development, 70*.

Pedersen, P. (1991b). Multiculturalism as a generic approach to counseling. *Journal of Counseling and Development, 70*(1), 6–12.

Pedersen, P. (1997). *Culture centered counseling interventions: Striving for accuracy*. Thousand Oaks, CA: Sage.

Pender, N. (1996). *Health promotion in nursing practice* (3rd ed.). Norwalk, CT: Appleton & Lange.

Peterson, J. (1993, April 11). Life in the United States, graded on a curve. *Los Angeles Times*, pp. A1, A16.

Pless, I., & Satterwhite, B. (1973). A measure of family functioning and its application. *Social Science & Medicine, 7*, 613–621.

Pope-Davis, D., & Coleman, H. (1997). *Multicultural counseling competencies*. Thousand Oaks, CA: Sage.

Pratt, L. (1976). *Family structure and effective health behavior: The energized family*. Boston: Houghton Mifflin.

Prinz, R., & Kent, R. (1978). Recording parent-adolescent interactions without the use of frequency or interval-by-interval coding. *Behavioral Therapy, 9*, 602–604.

Quinn, P., & Allen, K. (1989). Facing challenges and making compromises: How single mothers endure. *Family Relations, 38*, 390–395.

Ramey, C., & Ramey, S. (2000). *Quality child care and education: Evidence of lifelong and intergenerational benefits* (On-line). Available: http://www.cir.uab.edu/childcare/csbnews1.htm.

Reinhard, S. (1984). Perspective on the family's care-giving experience in mental illness. *Image, 26*(1), 71–78.

Reinhard, S., & Horwitz, A. (1995). Caregiver burden: Differentiating the content and consequences of family caregiving. *Journal of Marriage and the Family, 57*, 741–750.

Reitz, M., & Watson, K. (1992). *Adoption and the family*. New York: Guilford.

Richards, B. (1996). Gerontological family nursing. In S. Hanson & T. Boyd (Eds.), *Family health care nursing: Theory, practice, and research* (pp. 329–350). Philadelphia: Davis.

Riley, P., Sargent, G., Hartwell, S., & Patterson, J. (1997). Beyond law and ethics: An interdisciplinary course in family law and family therapy. *Journal of Marital and Family Therapy, 23*(4), 461–476.

Robinson, B. A. (2001, September 4). *Civil unions in Vermont*. Retrieved December 19, 2001, from Ontario Consultants on Religious Tolerance Web Site (online). Available: http://www.religioustolerance.org/hom_mar8.htm

Rolland, J. (1994a). *Families, illness and disability: An integrative treatment model*. New York: Basic Books.

Rolland, J. (1994b). In sickness and in health: The impact of illness on couples' relationships. *Journal of Marital and Family Therapy, 20*(4), 327–347.

Rose, L. (1996). Families of psychiatric patients. A critical review and future research directions. *Archives of Psychiatric Nursing, 10*, 67–74.

Rosenkoetter, M. (1991). Health promotion: The influence of pets on life patterns in the home. *Holistic Nursing Practice, 5*(2), 42–51.

Ross, B., & Cobb, K. (1990). *Family nursing: A nursing process approach*. Redwood, CA: Addison-Wesley.

Ross, C., Mirowsky, H., & Goldstein, D. (1990). The impact of the family on health: The decade in review. *Journal of Marriage and the Family, 52*, 1059–1078.

Ryan, D., & Carr, A. (2001). A study of differential effects of Tomm's questioning style on therapeutic alliance. *Family Process, 40*(1), 67–77.

Saluter, A., & Lugaila, T. (1998). *Marital status and living arrangements: March 1996*. U.S. Department of Commerce, Census Bureau, Current Population Reports, Population Characteristics, P20-496, pp. 1–6.

Sameroff, A., & Fiese, B. (1990). Transactional regulation and early interventions. In S. Micelles & J. Shonkoff (Eds.), *Handbook of early childhood intervention* (pp. 119–150). New York: Cambridge University Press.

Sayles-Cross, S. (1993). Perceptions of familial caregivers of elder adults. *Image, 15*(2), 88–96.

Scharff, D., & Scharff, J. (1991). *Objects relations family therapy*. Northvale, NJ: Jason Aronson.

Seaburn, D. (2001). Chronic illness. *Clinical Update, 3*(4), 1–6.

Shepard, M., & Mahon, M. (1996). Chronic conditions in the family. In P. Jackson & J. Vessey (Eds.), *Primary care of the child with a chronic condition* (2nd ed., pp. 41–46). St. Louis: Mosby.

Silverstein, D., & Demick, J. (1994). Toward an organizational-relational mode of open adoption. *Family Process, 33*(2), 111–124.

Slater, S. (1995). *The lesbian family life cycle*. New York: The Free Press.

Sluzki, C. (1974). On training to think interactionally. *Social Science and Medicine, 8*, 483–485.

Smilkstein, G. (1978). The Family APGAR: A proposal for a family function test and its use by physicians. *The Journal of Family Practice, 6* (6), 1231–1239.

Snowden, L., & Holschuh, J. (1992). Ethnic differences in emergency psychiatric care and hospitalization in a program for the severely mentally ill. *Journal of Community Mental Health, 28*, 281–291.

Spector, R. (1996). *Cultural diversity in health and illness* (4th ed.). Norwalk, CT: Appleton & Lange.

Stahl, S. (1998). Basic psychopharmacology of antidepressants. Part I. Antidepressants have seven distinct mechanisms of action. *Journal of Clinical Psychiatry, 59* (*suppl 4*), 5–14.

Stanhope, M., & Lancaster, J. (1996). *Community health nursing* (4th ed). St. Louis, MO: Mosby-Year Book.

Stanton, D. (1981). Strategic approaches to family therapy. In A. Gurman & D. Kniskern (Eds.), *Handbook of family therapy* (1st ed., pp. 361–402). New York: Brunner/Mazel.

Starfield, B. (1992). Child and adolescent health status measures. In Center for the Future of Children, *The future of children, 2*(2), 24–39. Los Altos, CA: The David and Lucile Packard Foundation.

State, M., Lombroso, P., Pauls, D., & Leckman, J. (2000). The genetics of childhood psychiatric disorders: A decade of progress. *Journal of the American Academy of Child and Adolescent Psychiatry, 39,* 946–962.

Steinberg, M. (2000, December/2001, January). Recognizing dissociative symptoms and its relevance to family therapists. *Family Therapy News,* 30–31.

Stone, R., Cafferata, G., & Sangl, J. (1987). Caregivers of the frail elderly: A national profile. *Gerontologist, 27,* 616–626.

Strong, B., & DeVault, C. (1993). *Essentials of marriage and family experience.* St. Paul, MN: West.

Sue, D. (1988). Psychotherapy services for ethnic minorities: Two decades of research findings. *American Psychologist, 43,* 301–308.

Sue, D., Arredondo, P., & McDavis, R. (1992). Multicultural competencies/standards: A pressing need. *Journal of Counseling and Development, 70*(4), 477–486.

Sue, D., Carter, R., Casa, J., Fouad, N., Ivey, A., Jensen, M., LaFromboise, T., Manese, J., Ponterotto, J., & Vazquez-Nutall, E. (1998). *Multicultural counseling competencies—Individual and organizational development.* Thousand Oaks, CA: Sage.

Sue, D., Fujino, D., Hu, L., Takeuchi, D., & Zane, N. (1991). Community mental health services for ethnic minority groups: A test of the cultural responsiveness hypothesis. *Journal of Counseling and Clinical Psychology, 59,* 433–540.

Sue, D., Ivey, A., & Pedersen, P. (1996). *A theory of multicultural counseling and therapy.* Pacific Grove, CA: Brooks/Cole.

Sue, D., & Sue, D. (1990). *Counseling the culturally different: Theory and practice* (2nd ed.). New York: John Wiley.

Sugar, M. (1992a, May). *Adolescents and their reactions to disaster.* Paper presented at the annual meeting of the American Society for Adolescent Psychiatry, San Francisco, CA.

Sugar, M. (1992b). Disasters. In M. Levine, W. Cary, A. Crocker (Eds.), *Developmental-behavioral pediatrics* (pp. 178–181). Philadelphia: Saunders.

Swanson, J., & Niles, M. (1997). *Community health nursing.* Philadelphia: Saunders.

Tallman, I. (1970). The family as a small problem solving group. *Journal of Marriage and the Family, 32,* 94–104.

Tinkham, G., & Voorhies, E. (1984). *Community health nursing—Evolution and process* (2nd ed.). New York: Appleton-Century-Crofts.

Tomm, K. (1987). Interventive interviewing. Part II: Reflexive questioning as a means to self healing. *Family Process, 26*(2), 167–183.

Tomm, K. (1988). Interventive interviewing. Part III: Intending to ask linear, circular, strategic, or reflexive questions? *Family Process, 27*(1), 1–15.

Tomm, K., & Lannamann, J. (1988, September/October). Questions as interventions. *The Family Therapy Networker,* 38–41.

Touliatos, J., Perlmutter, B., & Straus, A. (1990). *Handbook of family measurement techniques.* Newbury Park, CA: Sage.

Umberson, D., & Gove, W. (1989). Parenthood and psychological well-being: Theory, measurement, and stage in the family life course. *Journal of Family Issues, 10,* 440–462.

U.S. Bureau of the Census. (1983). *1980 Census of population. General population characteristics* (Part 1, Unites States Summary PC 80-1-61). Washington, DC: U.S. Government Printing Office.

U.S. Bureau of the Census. (1989a). Current populations reports, Series P-250, No. 1018. *Projections of the population in the United States by age, sex, and race: 1988 to 2080.* Washington, DC: U.S. Government Printing Office.

U.S. Bureau of the Census. (1989b). Current populations reports, Series P-60, No. 163. *Poverty in the United States: 1987, and earlier report.* Washington, DC: U.S. Government Printing Office.

U.S. Bureau of the Census. (1989c). Current populations reports, Series P-23, No. 162. *Studies in marriage and the family.* Washington, DC: U.S. Government Printing Office.

U.S. Bureau of the Census. (1989d). Current populations reports, Series P-20, No. 445. *Marital status and living arrangements: March 1989.* Washington, DC: U.S. Government Printing Office.

U.S. Bureau of the Census. (1990). Current Population reports, Series P-20, No. 12B. *Marital status and living arrangements: March 1990.* Washington, DC: U.S. Government Printing Office.

U.S. Bureau of the Census. (1991a). Current populations reports, Series P-60, No. 173. *Child support and alimony: 1989.* Washington, DC: U.S. Government Printing Office.

U.S. Bureau of the Census. (1991b). Current populations reports, Series P-20, No. 461 *Marital status and living arrangements: March 1991.* Washington, DC: U.S. Government Printing Office.

U.S. Bureau of the Census. (1992a). Current populations reports, Series P-20, No. 458 *Household and family characteristics: 1991.* Washington, DC: U.S. Government Printing Office.

U.S. Bureau of the Census. (1992b). Current populations reports, Series P-23, No. 180. *Marriage, divorce and remarriage in the 1990s.* Washington, DC: U.S. Government Printing Office.

U.S. Bureau of the Census. (1992c). Current populations reports, Series P-20, No. 468. *Marriage status and living arrangements: March 1992.* Washington, DC: U.S. Government Printing Office.

U.S. Bureau of the Census. (1992d). Current populations reports, Series P-23, No. 181. *Households, families and children: A 30 year perspective.* Washington, DC: U.S. Government Printing Office.

U.S. Bureau of the Census. (1992e). *1990 Census of population. General population characteristics.* Washington, DC: U.S. Government Printing Office.

U.S. Bureau of the Census. (1995). *Sixty-five plus in the United States. Statistical brief.* Washington, DC: U.S. Department of Commerce, Economics, and Statistics Administration.

U.S. Bureau of the Census. (1997, October 3). Age, sex household relationship, race and Hispanic origin and selected statuses: Ratio of income to poverty level in 1996 (online). Available: http://ferret.bls.census.gov/macro/03197/pov/2_001-3.htm.

U.S. Bureau of the Census. (1998). Poverty: 1997 Highlights (online). Available: http://www.census.gov/hhes/poverty/poverty97/pov97hi.html.

U.S. Department of Health and Human Services. (1979). *Healthy people: The surgeon general's report on health promotion and disease prevention.* (U.S. Public Health Service, Pub. No. PHS 79-55071) Washington, DC: U.S. Government Printing Office.

U.S. Department of Health and Human Services. (1980). *Promoting health/Preventing disease: Objectives for the nation.* Washington, DC: U.S. Government Printing Office.

U.S. Department of Health and Human Services. (1990). *Healthy people 2000: National health promotion and disease prevention objectives* (Department of Health and Human Services, Office of Public Health and Science). Washington, DC: U.S. Government Printing Office.

U.S. Department of Health and Human Services. (1995). *Psychosocial issues for children and families in disasters—A guide for primary care physicians* (Public Health Service, Substance Abuse and Mental Health Services Administration, Center for Mental Health Services with the Federal Emergency Management Agency-Interagency Agreement Number- 93-IA-MH-84-08). Washington, DC: National Mental Health Services Knowledge Exchange.

U.S. Department of Health and Human Services. (1998). *Healthy people 2010: National health promotion and disease prevention objectives* (Department of Health and Human Services, Publication No. PHS 91-50213). Washington, DC: U.S. Government Printing Office.

U.S. Department of Justice, Office of Justice Programs, Office of Juvenile Justice and Delinquency Prevention. (2001, June). *Healthy families America—Fact sheet #23.* Washington, DC: Author. (www.healthyfamiliesamerica.org)

van der Kolk, B., Perry, J., & Herman, J. (1991). Childhood origins of self-destructive behavior. *American Journal of Psychiatry, 148,* 1665–1671.

Venters, M. (1986). Family life and cardiovascular risk: Implications for the prevention of chronic disease. *Social Science and Medicine, 22,* 1067–1074.

Visher, E., & Visher, J. (1996). *Therapy with stepfamilies.* New York: Brunner/Mazel.

Voydanoff, P., & Donnelly, S. (1988). Economic distress, family coping and quality of family life. In P. Voydanoff & L. Le Majka (Eds.), *Families and economic distress* (pp. 97–115). Newbury Park, CA: Sage.

Wachtel, E. (1982). The family psyche over three generations. The genogram revisited. *Journal of Marital and Family Therapy, 8,* 335–343.

Walker, T. (1992). Family law in the fifty states: An overview. *Family Law Quarterly, 25,* 417–515.

Walker, A., Pratt, C., & Oppy, N. (1992). Perceived reciprocity in family caregiving. *Family Relations, 41,* 82–85.

Walsh, F. (1993). Conceptualization of normal family processes. In F. Walsh (Ed.), *Normal family processes* (2nd ed., pp. 3–69). New York: Guilford.

White, M., & Epston, D. (1980). *Narrative means to therapeutic ends*. New York: Norton.

Wisensale, S. (1993). State and federal initiatives in family policy. In T. H. Brubaker (Ed.), *Family relations: Challenges for the future* (pp. 229–250). Newbury Park, CA: Sage.

Wolff, E. (1995). How the pie is sliced: America's growing concentration of wealth. *The American Prospect, 22*, 58–64.

Wright, L., & Leahey, M. (1990). Trends in the nursing of families. *Journal of Advanced Nursing, 15*, 148–154.

Wright, L., & Leahey, M. (1994). *Nurses and families. A guide to family assessment and intervention* (2nd ed.). Philadelphia: Davis.

Wright, L., & Leahey, M. (2000). *Nurses and families. A guide to family assessment and intervention* (3rd ed.). Philadelphia: F. A. Davis.

Wright, L., Watson, W., & Bell, J. (1990). The family nursing unit: A unique integration of research, education and clinical practice. In J. Bell, W. Watson, & L. Wright (Eds.), *The cutting edge of family nursing* (pp. 95–112). Calgary, Alberta: Family Nursing Unit Publications.

Zimmerman, S. (1992). *Family policies and family well-being: The role of political culture*. Newbury Park, CA: Sage.

Index

About the Contributors

HARLENE ANDERSON is the director and a founding member of the Houston Galveston Institute in Houston, Texas. She is known internationally as a teacher and consultant for her work in forging links between postmodern theory and collaborative clinical practice.

RUTH P. COX is Associate Professor of Nursing in the School of Nursing graduate program at the University of Alabama, Birmingham. She is a licensed marriage and family therapist and supervisor, an advanced registered nurse practitioner in mental health, a family nurse practitioner, and a certified trauma specialist.

KEN FARR is a clinical nurse specialist in adult psychiatric/mental health nursing with a subspecialization in geriatric/psychiatric nursing. He is employed in a teaching role at the University of Alabama at Birmingham School of Nursing in Birmingham. His work experience includes working in private practice with hospital privileges and being a consultant to several nursing homes.

BEVERLY HOGAN is a clinical nurse specialist in adult psychiatric/mental health nursing. She is employed in a teaching role at the University of Alabama at Birmingham School of Nursing in Birmingham. She has worked in a community health center and has been director of education in a public psychiatric hospital.

NORM KELTNER is a professor at the University of Alabama at Birmingham School of Nursing, Birmingham. His clinical work centers around the psychobiology of the brain and psychotropic medications with extensive publications in this area.

SYLVIA LONDON is a professor and supervisor in the Master's in Family Therapy and Social Constructionism program at the National University of Mexico, School of Psychology, in Mexico City. She is co-founder of Grupo

Campos Eliseos. Irma Punsky and Conchita Quiroz are supervisors in the Master's in Family Therapy and Social Constructionism program at the National University of Mexico, School of Psychology, and Rocio Martinez Zaid and Alberto Díaz are students in the program.

EDDIE PARRISH is a marriage and family therapist who works as a family minister with his local church in Baton Rouge, LA. He has been an associate professor in the Marriage and Family Therapy program at Abilene Christian College in Abilene, TX.